Reviewers all over the c̲o̲—  ̲—
DOM OF SEXUAL LOVE.

"The key word in this v̲—
dom to be human and l̲—
husband and wife. It is a̲—
be married, for it examin̲— ̲—ᵤᵤ psychological elements in human ̲—̲y." *Marriage*

"By delicately interweaving the physical, psychological, and
spiritual dimensions of human sexuality, the Birds beautifully
describe what is at once a physical act, a sanctifying union, and
a spiritual experience wrapped into one by a truly human and
Christian love that is infinitely more than mere 'sex technique,'
which, however, they also treat candidly." *Extension*

". . . the discussion is complete, detailed, frank and reverent,
and will clear away many doubts, disagreements and misconceptions that mar and cause unnecessary suffering in many marriages." *Today's Family*

"THE FREEDOM OF SEXUAL LOVE should be read by every
Christian—lover, newlywed, parent, teenager." *The Observer*

"A subject that is often shied away from is here treated with
candor and sensitivity by a husband-wife team highly qualified
for the job: Dr. Bird is a clinical psychologist and psychotherapist who has written widely on the matter; Lois F. Bird is his
wife and the mother of nine children." *Review for Religious*

"This book is for everybody. It is for people about to marry,
for married couples to grow on, for parents to aid them in developing healthy knowledge and respect for sex in their children, and for religious and those wishing to become religious.
By better understanding the world of their lay friends they can
better understand their own world. THE FREEDOM OF SEXUAL
LOVE, in fact, uniquely qualifies for a kind of spiritual reading
—something few books can offer." *St. Louis Review*

THE FREEDOM OF
SEXUAL LOVE

JOSEPH W. BIRD
and
LOIS F. BIRD

IMAGE BOOKS

A DIVISION OF DOUBLEDAY & COMPANY, INC.

GARDEN CITY, NEW YORK

Image Book edition 1970
by special arrangement with Doubleday & Company, Inc.
Image Books edition published September 1970

Nihil Obstat: John A. Goodwine, J.C.D.
Censor Librorum

Imprimatur: ✠ Terence J. Cooke, D.D., V.G.
Archdiocese of New York
December 14, 1966

The nihil obstat and imprimatur are official declarations that a book or pamphlet is free of doctrinal or moral error. No implication is contained therein that those who have granted the nihil obstat and imprimatur agree with the contents, opinions or statements expressed.

To our children—

Paul, Ann, Susan, Kathleen, Joan, Stephen, Michael, Mary, and Diane.

You have given us far more than we can hope to repay. Through you we have learned much of the meaning of love. And through you our oneness has grown. We can never be worthy of such a gift.

ACKNOWLEDGMENTS

THERE ARE so many to whom we are indebted, far too many to list. But we remain in their debt and they remain in our prayers. There are a few, however, toward whom we are especially grateful for the gifts they have given us through their insights, influence, and suggestions both in our marriage and in the writing of this book: Reverend Fathers William Cane, Paul Caringella, John C. Desmond, James Mara S.J., Daniel C. O'Connell S.J., and Victor Wilkiemeyer.

We owe many thanks to Mr. Clayton C. Barbeau whose prodding started us on the manuscript, whose encouragement eased our doubts and hesitations, and whose expert advice did much to pave the way.

We feel that much has been added to what we hoped to say in this book through the Foreword so generously written by Monsignor J. D. Conway. We are deeply grateful to him.

Mr. John J. Delaney, our editor at Doubleday & Company, must be given a special thank you. His suggestions have repeatedly made such good sense that we have been embarrassed at not having thought of them ourselves.

And for her patience under what must have developed

into pressure, we want to thank our typist, Miss Marilyn Kampfen.

And to "our couples," those husbands and wives who have permitted us to share in the growth of their marriage: our gratitude and our love, always.

FOREWORD

OUR CATHOLIC CONCEPTS of marriage have probably changed more in the past forty years than they had in the previous nineteen centuries. The change has not been a reversal but an expansion of vision and a deepening of understanding; it is that growth of perception, inspired and guided by the Holy Spirit, which represents a true development of doctrine. Two human factors have contributed greatly to this growth. First, laymen experienced in the realities of marriage have contributed a new empirical dimension to our thought; and secondly, we have experienced a growing awareness of the human person, of his dignity and integrity.

Our new sensitivity to the human person in his totality tends to break our ancient habit of viewing him in conceptual compartments. We are concerned with the total growth of his personality, and we realize the futility of trying to measure or guide that growth by isolated norms of biology or psychology. Man's growth as a person takes place in a definite sociological and economic situation. Education plays a vital role; health is important; motive forces must be understood; and neither genetics nor demography can be ignored.

When we try to see the human person in total perspec-

tive we realize that the predominant force which vitalizes
and integrates his true growth is love. As a person he
needs to love and to be loved; he must give love generously and receive it with confidence. And this love must
be interpersonal, whether between human persons or with
the three divine persons. Without this giving and receiving
of personal love man's growth is distorted.

Love was the basis of sanctity in the ancient law of
Moses: love of God and love of fellow man. "Listen, O
Israel; the Lord is our God, the Lord alone; so you must
love the Lord your God with all your mind and all your
heart and all your strength" (Deut. 6, 4–5). "You must
not avenge yourself, nor bear a grudge . . . but you must
love your neighbor as yourself" (Lev. 19, 19).

Love was stressed most forcibly by Jesus Christ in His
word and example, and the early Christians seem to have
understood it and practiced it. The world recognized them
by their love for one another.

But somewhere in the early centuries of Christianity
this vivid awareness of the sanctifying force of interpersonal love seems to have been lost. We find little trace of
it at the Council of Nicaea, and much less at Ephesus and
Chalcedon. Hermits sought sanctity by separating themselves from their fellow men, content to love their neighbors in fancy but not in fact. Monks sought sanctity in separating themselves from the world and often developed a
zeal for doctrine, true or false, which obscured their love
for their brethren.

And nowhere in Christian society did interpersonal love
seem to play a less important and less sanctifying role than
in marriage. Catholic teachings about marriage, from the
fifth century to the fifteenth, and even to our own time,
were dominated by the doctrine of St. Augustine. For him
the love between husband and wife involved too much
concupiscence to be sanctifying. Indeed this love could

hardly be expressed at all without some measure of sin. Only procreation justified intercourse; so the normal expression of marital love could not be lawful unless procreation were both possible and intended.

Augustine found three values in marriage: the good of children, the good of fidelity, and the good of the sacrament which made marriage permanent. But only the good of children justified intercourse, though fidelity might justify one partner in paying the debt to the other, as a remedy for concupiscence and to prevent greater evil.

Marriage was a status tolerated by God for the benefit of the human race. The husband and wife could hardly live in this status without sin. Indeed continence had a greater value than procreation; so the husband and wife who piously refrained from intercourse were more holy than those who sought children. Augustine did make passing mention of mutual companionship between the partners in marriage, but sanctifying love was never proposed by him as a value.

This rigid doctrine of Augustine was taught with no twinge of sympathy by the monks of the following centuries, and it received its most rigorous interpretation from Pope St. Gregory the Great. According to this influential Pontiff any pleasure taken in intercourse is a sin even though conception be possible. Married people befoul their intercourse by taking pleasure in it. However, if they intend to conceive a child by their act, their sin is not a great one and they can obtain forgiveness for it by frequent prayer.

St. Thomas Aquinas was able to find positive value in the joys of marriage, in theory. But he judged that in practice intercourse could hardly be devoid of sin because the intensity of its pleasures took away, for the moment, man's use of his highest faculty, reason.

It is hard to tell how deeply these teachings of theologians impressed themselves on the consciences of the Christian people, but medieval guides for confessors and some of the sermons preached during the late middle ages lead us to believe that the influence was often profound and possibly extensive. We do know that Jansenism, which became widely popular in the late seventeenth century greatly influenced the attitude of the Catholic people of Western Europe toward sexual morality until modern times. Those morals which we term Victorian were the formalized and decadent expression of the rigorous attitudes of Jansenism, Puritanism, and the Augustinian influences of the Reformation.

At no period prior to modern times has the Church positively proposed the marital life and the carnal love of husband and wife as means to great sanctity. It is hard to find a saint in the calendar who led a normal married life. Indeed I cannot think of a single one at the moment. St. Margaret of Scotland comes to mind, but she received news on her deathbed that her husband had been killed in battle; so she died a holy widow. Otherwise we would have to design a special Mass for her. We have no Mass for holy wives.

St. Thomas More might be cited as an example, but he had a long period of penance in the Tower of London, plus the blood of martyrdom, to purify him of the sins of marriage. Even at that it took him a long time to get canonized.

Our modern appreciation of the positive value of sexual love in marriage probably finds its first solid base in the moral theology of St. Alphonsus Liguori, who lived during most of the eighteenth century. We look back on him as a rigorist, a legalist, and a casuist, but in his own day he was considered dangerously lax, an opponent of legal formalism. He was certainly a potent antidote to Jansenism.

Alphonsus seems to have been the first to see in marital

intercourse a legitimate outlet for sexual desire. It was a proper remedy for concupiscence. The purpose of obtaining pleasure was a legitimate reason for marrying, though it was an extrinsic and accidental end of marriage, like solidifying inheritances or conciliating feuds between families.

Modern thinking on this subject really began with Dietrich von Hildebrand, a professor of philosophy at the University of Munich, and the first married layman to be accepted as an authority on the subject of Catholic marriage. About 1925 he began to teach and write on the positive value of marital intercourse for the husband and wife, as an expression and fulfillment of their love for each other; "it participates after a certain fashion in the sacramental meaning of matrimony." It is an expression of marital fidelity which requires that person meet person in a giving of self. There is something sacred and sanctifying about it.

A few years later, Herbort Doms, a priest, scientist, philosopher and theologian, gave a sound theological basis to the ideas of Hildebrand, and pointed out the biological errors which had distorted earlier evaluations of the sexual act. He also enriched the concept of the marital relationship by viewing it in the light of personalism: a giving of one person to another, the fulfillment of one person in another, the spiritual giving of self in joy, love, and abandonment.

These ideas did not meet with immediate acceptance, but about thirty years later the Fathers of Vatican Council II endorsed the following statements in their Constitution on the Church in the Modern World:

"Thus a man and a woman, who by their compact of conjugal love 'are no longer two, but one flesh' (Matt. 19, 6), render mutual help and service to each other through an intimate union of their persons and their actions. Through this union they experience the meaning of their oneness and attain to it with growing perfection day by day . . ."

"Christ the Lord abundantly blessed this many-faceted love, welling up as it does from the fountain of divine love . . . Authentic married love is caught up into divine love and is governed and enriched by Christ's redeeming power and the saving activity of the Church . . . This love is an eminently human one since it is directed from one person to another through an affection of the will; it involves the good of the whole person, and therefore can enrich the expressions of body and mind with a unique dignity, ennobling these expressions as special ingredients and signs of the friendship distinctive of marriage . . . Such love, merging the human with the divine, leads the spouses to a free and mutual gift of themselves . . . The actions within marriage by which the couple are united intimately and chastely are noble and worthy ones. Expressed in a manner which is truly human, these actions promote the mutual self-giving by which spouses enrich each other . . ."

The Fathers are restrained in their words, but they make it clear that the human, sexual love of spouses for each other is good and sanctifying. It is in conformity with this spirit of Vatican II that Joseph and Lois Bird have written their own love story, offering to others the benefits of their experiences and their insights. It is evident that they consider love-making an art to be learned and taught, an art which expresses truth in a manner which is authentic and designed to provoke a comprehending and inspired response.

The man who truly loves his wife will not be content with crude, instinctive expressions of his love. He will seek expressions which elicit love at the same time they give assurance of it, which will make love grow and become more profound, more personal, more all-embracing. And he will not confine his art to moments of intense sexual involvement; he will work at it all day, every day.

A book like this would not have received Catholic approval a few years ago. Many of us recall a book of premarital sex instructions co-authored by a priest and a doctor, written with respect and dignity, which was banned by high Church authority less than two decades ago. And since that time I have found nothing to take its needed place until this volume of *The Freedom of Sexual Love*. Books of sex instructions and the art of making love weigh down the shelves of most book stores, but they lack the spiritual tone, the integrated wholesomeness, and the authentic morality of this book.

Most books on marriage written by Catholic authors either avoid any frank treatment of the subject of sex, or handle it as a problem in moral theology. Joseph and Lois Bird treat it as an integral part of their own fruitful, happy, and holy life, on the basis of expert knowledge and experience in psychology, and in conjunction with prayer.

It was my privilege to be pastor of the Bird family at one time, and my dominant memory regarding them is the decorous and diligent attention of the Bird children lined up in the front pew at Mass. Psychologists are reputed to be permissive, but I doubt that the Bird children would endorse this reputation.

MONSIGNOR J. D. CONWAY

CONTENTS

THE FREEDOM OF SEXUAL LOVE

INTRODUCTION

THIS IS A love story. It is the story of sexual love, the love of man and woman united in the mystery of a sacrament which joins them in one flesh. It is an attempt to examine the physical, emotional, and spiritual meaning of the marital embrace. In this, we can never fully succeed since our subject matter is an encounter, and a relationship, so profound, so complex, and so enriched with grace that it has been called "a glimpse of the Beatific Vision."

Tragically, it has also been called the foremost cause of marital discord.

Within context, both descriptions are probably valid. They represent the difference between the ideal and what many have found as their reality; the difference between what marriage can, and should, become, and what it too frequently fails to become.

Surveys of psychotherapists and marriage counselors, reports from social agencies, and articles written by physicians and lawyers, all put *sex* at the head of the problem list. It has been cited as the primary cause of divorce. But is *sex* really the problem? Does so-called "sexual incompatibility" deserve to be called the leading destroyer of marriages? Yes and no. To be sure, many couples complain of sexual difficulties. Furthermore, many complain that such problems are the major disruptive factor in their marriage. Most authorities, however, would be quick to point out that these difficulties are usually only symptoms of more global conflict between the spouses. Sexual love is always reflective of the total love in the marriage; hence, if the couple complain of sexual troubles, it is the total marriage which is in trouble, and the total marriage which is most probably deficient in love. There are, of course, some cases in which sexual conflicts evidence deeper emotional problems of either, or both, husband or wife. But in any case, when we speak of sexual incompatibility it is nearly always a symptom we are talking about rather than the basic problem.

There are also many couples who have essentially sound Christian marriages. They are not tearing each other to shreds in rivalry and bitterness. Nor are they tortured neurotics. They relate to each other in ways which express love and affection. Usually, they think of their marriage as happy; seldom do they complain of sexual difficulties. In fact, if one were to suggest that they might have a sexual problem, they would probably deny it with conviction. And yet, something is lacking. Without being aware of it, they too have failed to find sexual love. They have failed to achieve that complete unity which is the distinguishing characteristic of a Christian marriage. Although it may never erupt in conflict, their sexual relationship is *not good!* It has not matured and it has ceased growing. It has not become, as it should, a source of deep satisfaction and fulfillment drawing them ever closer. In sexual love, they're standing still. Blocked in the development of their sexual love by lack of information, misinformation, or unhealthy attitudes, the total growth in their marriage has been arrested. It is to them we address this love story. Most of all, to them.

We read much today about sexual "liberation," the so-called "new freedom." Sunday supplements, college news-papers, and slick-paper periodicals provide a ready market for those writing of the "new morality." But liberation *from* what? And *to* what? In our sexually "free" society, freedom has become enslavement; liberation has become license. Sexuality is increasingly discussed, and yet its meaning seems increasingly obscured.

This confusion has affected many Christian couples, far more than many might guess. The result of it, we can only describe as tragic. The fact that they are Christian, and are struggling to perfect themselves in Christian mar-riage while living under such a cloud of confusion and doubt, makes it even more a tragedy. The goal toward which they are striving, fulfillment in Christ through their marriage, seems most of the time so far away. It doesn't help to tell them that sexual adjustment must be achieved if the marriage is to succeed. They are trying to discover the splendor of sexual love. They have heard what it can become and they want to find it. But instead, they find only sexual problems.

In spite of what some "sex experts" say, the solution will not be found in physical adjustments or techniques. Such an approach is far too narrow. The dimensions of human sexuality are physical, psychological, and spiritual, and to stress one to the exclusion of the others is a serious error, and one which may be detrimental. And yet there are scores of books and articles on marital love with just such singular approaches.

A number of secular marriage manuals instruct in a wide variety of physical techniques, acts, and positions, but little else. These how-to-do-it books promise marital bliss; all the readers need do is practice these various phys-ical skills. All well and good, except it doesn't work. We have seen far too many couples attempt such a method to remedy their sexual problems only to find that human beings are more than mere physical machines.

And then there are the popularizers of psychoanalytic concepts. Everything to them is a manifestation of unconscious drives. They throw out love, replace it with the Id, and they preach a hard-core determinism which strips man of his humanity and makes human sexuality a mere outlet for the libido. Above all, they reject morality in sex. For the most part, they misinterpret Freud, but no matter, they all too often find ready acceptance for their pseudo-psychology.

Christian writers, on the other hand, have often gone astray in the opposite direction. In writing of marriage, they often avoid any explicit treatment of its physical aspects. They give it no more than a passing nod of acceptance but seem either unable or unwilling to deal with what they term man's baser nature. Hence, they set up an abnormal dichotomy of mind and body or spirit and flesh. And human beings, as human beings, cease to exist in these writings.

Many couples do lack information, but if the problem is only a lack of information, the harm is slight and the remedy is obvious. Seldom is it this simple. In searching for the cause of sexual difficulties, we must probe all areas of human existence. Solutions will not be found in merely learning techniques. They will not be found in pietistic essays which avoid the subject (and thus, by implication, view it as *bad*). And they most certainly won't be found in "liberating" society from moral restraint and the obligation to love.

Not that a liberation is not needed. It is. But in the way in which many bring sexuality "out in the open," something is left behind. That something is *love*. It is love which gives sexuality its beauty, which gives it purpose. And it is love which makes it a sanctifying act. While it is a physical *act,* it is transcended through mutual love and becomes a spiritual *experience.* If it is to have any meaning, the two are inseparable. Those who emphasize the physical aspects but ignore or deny the spiritual, find only a hollow shell of marital love; they are left wandering in the emptiness and boredom of an egocentric world. On the other hand, any failure to recognize or gratefully accept the physical aspects of marriage and all they imply, can scar the marriage as deeply. In effect it denies the meaning of the sacrament and disparages the means God has given for the greatest expression of human love. Holding either view can have nothing but a pernicious effect on the marriage.

It would be comforting to think that sex education would solve these problems, but, as it is usually given, it is seldom enough. Having acquired some knowledge of the physical aspects, the couple may go no further. But unless they do, their sexual relationship will remain fixated at the level of sensualism. Or merely anatomy. What is needed, but seldom given, is an education in sexual *love.* There is only one way, however, that this can be communicated: it must be *witnessed.* Even in our age of sexual candor, many are pitifully ignorant. And yet they don't know know where to turn for answers. Or they are too embarrassed to ask the questions.

Those who might help them, couples who can witness truly rewarding marriages, are often strangely silent. They have found Christ in their marriage and yet they hide this light under a bushel of secrecy and defend their silence with clichés about "privacy" and "sanctity of the home." How then are they witnessing their vocation? And how are they meeting the obligations of their apostolate?

Recently, at a meeting of a group formed to study the meaning of Christian marriage, marital sexuality was sug-

gested as a topic. The members, however, dismissed it in
short order. By vote, they decided it wasn't a proper area
for discussion. If this is representative, where are young
couples to look for answers? We can say that they should
have been taught by their parents, but what if they were
not?

We have called this a love story. We hope that the
reader will find in it a story of love. It is our attempt to
witness. We have tried at all times to be candid and explicit. Such candor, we recognize, may offend some. Perhaps this is unavoidable, although regrettable, since if we
are to attempt to answer the questions we are asked, frank-
ness and clarity are essential. The various aspects of sexuality which we discuss arise from the questions asked by
many married couples. We hope that we may help clear
away some of their confusion regarding Christian sexuality
as it is lived; and this demands candor. Furthermore, in
freely and openly writing of the experience of sexual love
in Christian marriage, we hope to convey our deep convictions that this experience is a very beautiful and sanctifying expression of love; and we simply cannot be reticent
or evasive if we are to witness such love.

In the marital union are to be found the mystery and
the meaning of Christian marriage. The sexual love of
husband and wife is the witnessing sign of their vocation.
But in order to live this vocation, they each must be free
to give and receive love and emotionally free to accept
the gift of their sexuality and to find in it a reflection of
God's love. Many are not. They may be painfully aware
of the sexual responsibilities of marriage, but the fact that
their awareness is painful is, itself, often an indication
that they lack understanding of both the rewards it offers
as well as the scope of these obligations. Various factors
may contribute to this inability to love and be loved. They
may suffer from moral doubts, socially reinforced inhibitions, or crippling fears, but in any case they are blind

to the joy of sexual love and hence, for them, marital love becomes, at best, solely an obligation in justice, at worst, a torture.

This need not be. Such husbands and wives can change. They can find that their marriage need not be an endless succession of disillusionments and frustrations. They can begin to grow together rather than apart. If they accept the redemptive grace promised in the sacrament which unites them, they will find the motivation to love. They then must learn how best to love—each other. This will often be a difficult struggle since loving may demand so much; our own selfish desires tend always to get in the way. But it can be done. The answers are there and they can be found. By looking outside of ourselves to those we are trying to love, we can discover the ways to love. By looking inside of ourselves, we can uncover the barriers which block our loving.

This book is neither a marriage manual nor a fledgling theology of sex. It is intended as an expression of marital love *as it is lived*. It has been "our book," and now it is yours. In writing it, we have drawn upon a number of sources. We are especially indebted to those individuals, single and married, clergy and laity, who have opened the doors of their lives to us. The final responsibility, however, is ours alone. Our primary source throughout has been the marriage we have lived and are living. For the love God has shown us through each other, and for the graces with which He has surrounded us, we are humbly grateful, and more than awed. With His help, perhaps we can share this gift. Our prayer is that others, the clergy, seeking to understand this sacramental vocation, the unmarried, struggling to prepare themselves for it, and the married, striving to live it, may come to find what we have continually rediscovered: that the marital union is a commitment in love and a channel of grace through which husband and wife find Christ.

CHAPTER I

Promise of Eden

Then the Lord God said, "It is not good that the man is alone; I will make him a helper like himself" (Gen. 2:18).

Our first parents *knew* the meaning of sexuality. And they knew its beauty, and its holiness. The Creator had blessed their union and revealed His plan for it. Their sexual love, God said, was not merely good, it was very good. This, He revealed to them, was to be a total commitment, one of love, a human love transcending all others. And its highest beauty was to be found in the sexual embrace.

Then the man said, "She now is bone of my bone, and flesh of my flesh; she shall be called Woman, for from man she has been taken." For this reason a man leaves his father and mother, and clings to his wife, and the two become one flesh (Gen. 2:23–24).

Imagine, if you will, the perfect honeymoon: an idyllic setting, trees, flowers, flowing rivers, complete privacy, and the ideal couple—just made for each other, with no cares or worries, and the promise of a lifetime of happiness. This bride and groom begin their marriage with a complete understanding of their relationship; their attitudes toward sex and love, their concepts of manhood and womanhood, are all wholesome; they have been taught no distorted views which must be unlearned in a painful adjustment. And lastly, picture such a honeymoon never ending, only increasing in joy and growing in beauty each day.

This was Eden. This was the way God intended it, the manner in which He gave the gift of sexual love to man and woman. No false modesty, no twisted inhibitions, only the purity of love. *Both the man and his wife were naked, but they felt no shame* (Gen. 2 : 25). This was the way it was; and this was the way it was to remain. Marriage: a continual honeymoon.

But it didn't last. Adam and his wife were tempted, and fell. And the honeymoon came to an end.

The story we read of this honeymoon is brief, no more than a paragraph. But what can be said of such total happiness? As in the daily newspapers, strife, trouble, and unhappiness make copy, but seldom do we find much to say of happiness. It is a state of balance, of peace, without cares or conflict. Hence, to state that we are happy is to imply that we have found an absence of all those conditions which cause us to feel pain, tension, and a sense of loss. Happiness, like love, is inclusive. Once we say, "They were happy," we have said everything.

After the fall, however, all the evils destructive of happiness erupted. Man and woman were evicted from their honeymoon garden. They found pain, disappointment, drudgery, and the dark night of sin. Before the fall, the relationship between the original man and woman, the archetype of all future marriage, was one of perfect equality and love. He greeted her creation with gratitude and joy. Now he was no longer alone; he had *"a mate of his own kind"* (Gen. 2 : 18). They were joined as *one*. The words he spoke in accepting the gift of his bride showed a realization of the character of this union: It was monog-

amous; it was indissoluble; and it was a total commitment
of self to another. This was to be the ideal of marriage,
the ideal of human love. In the darkness which followed
the fall, man did not lose his knowledge of the ideal, but in
the mist in which he waited agonizingly for the promised
Messiah, the ideal was obscured.

Sexual love, in the accounts of the Old Testament,
seemed often very far from loving. The emphasis was on
the procreative function of sexuality, and not infrequently
to the exclusion of love. The ideal of monogamy was re-
laxed; polygamy, as well as concubinage, was condoned.
Abraham, for example, at the bidding of his wife, Sarah,
had a child by Agar, Sarah's maid. This apparently was
not an exceptional case. Jacob, for instance, loved Rachael
enough to work several years for his future father-in-law in
order to win her in marriage, and yet not only did he take
a second wife, Rachael's sister, Lia, but, like Abraham, he
had a child by his wife's servant girl. Continuation of the
species was considered a value transcending all others.
Women, for that matter, were valued for their ability to
bear children, but little else, and a wife could feel secure
and confident of her husband's love only if she bore him a
son (cf. Gen. 29 : 32). No longer were they recognized as
the equal of man; rather, they were viewed more as indentured servants, or even chattels, to be bought and sold,
taken and disposed of. Man had strayed a long way from
Eden. Even when human love was mentioned, as in the
story of David and Michol (1 Kings 18 : 20–27), it was seldom tied to the ideal of monogamy (he took two other
wives and a number of concubines), nor fidelity (he committed adultery with Bethsabee, had a child by her, and
arranged to have her husband killed [2 Kings 11 : 2–27]).

Polygamy, adultery, incest, rape, and sexual perversion
are woven throughout the Old Testament. After glimpsing
the heights of Eden, we are shown the depths to which

sexuality fell in the fallen state. The thread of beauty and
the promise were retained, however, illuminated by mo-
mentary flashes of light. Prophetic couples, witnessing the
ideal, formed the bridge between the Eden that was lost
and the Eden that was promised. Step by step the events
of the Old Testament led toward that moment when the
doors would open and man would step out of the darkness and into the light of the New Jerusalem. The chaste
love of Tobias and Sara (Tob. 6 : 18; 8 : 4–8) formed
such a marriage. Mutual love in God, sanctified by prayer,
bound them together. Once again, the ideal was that of
Eden. Their marriage was a union of equality; it was
monogamous, indissoluble—and transcending.

The ideal of human—sexual—love was retained also in
another way. The relationship of God and His people was
described by the Old Testament writers in terms of human
love. Jahweh was pictured as the lover, His people the beloved. This tradition was followed by Isaias (5 : 1–7;
54 : 4–8), Jeremias (2 : 2; 2 : 32), and Ezechiel (16; 23).
The covenant between the Lord and Israel was described
as a marriage, and the idolatry of Israel was seen by Osee
as adultery (1 : 2–8).

In exquisite poetic form, the love of God for His bride,
Israel, and the love which she returns is portrayed in the
prose of the Canticle of Canticles. Here, in the lyric words
of sexual love, is painted the picture of the perfect bride
and the perfect marriage. The bride is the ideal Israel, led
to perfection through mutual love and growing in love
toward a spiritual union with her groom, God.

The "greatest of songs" is also an inspired portrayal of
the ideal of sexual love. Here is God drawing man again
to the honeymoon of Eden with all the depth and sacredness intended in the marital union.

The human love of the Canticle of Canticles and the
marriage of Tobias and Sara, viewed in the context of the

Old Testament, however, seem almost unreal, as if only a dream. And it was a dream—and a promise. The Law did not demand such a standard. Only with the New Covenant, the fulfillment of the ancient law, was it fully restored. Christian writers have traditionally interpreted the Canticle of Canticles in terms of the union of Christ and His Church. And in this metaphor, the perfection of Christian marriage is portrayed in all its intended glory. Before the coming of the Messiah, polygamy and divorce had both been permitted to exist as a recognition of the hardness of heart of the people (Matt. 19 : 8). But when Christ spoke of marriage, He spoke in the words of the ideal set forth in the Creation: *"Have you not read that the Creator, from the beginning, made them male and female, and said, 'For this cause a man shall leave his father and mother, and cleave to his wife, and the two shall become one flesh?' Therefore now they are no longer two, but one flesh. What therefore God has joined together, let no man put asunder"* (Matt. 19 : 4–6). Thus Christ, the second Adam, brought man, in the union of marriage, full circle, fulfilling the prophecies and the Law, returning to it the beauty and mystery proclaimed by the first Adam.

Love was to be the new law, the *Law of Christ* (Gal. 6 : 2). Such human love is not easily understood. Being a human love which reflects a divine love, it must remain a "great mystery." It is a mystery which is rooted deep in the mystery of God and in our acceptance, in faith, of the Trinity. And it is rooted in the mystery of Christ's redemptive love for His Church.

As the perfection of love, the Father gives Himself totally to His Son. Perfect union is achieved in this giving. All of the identity and being of the Father are given to the Son without reservation. Hence, the Second Person of the Trinity is the Word of the Father. He, also, has the completion of the Divine Nature; He is True God.

Human love is the striving for such union with another; it is the lovers' desire to "become one." Such completeness is not to be ours, however. It will be found only in God. Hence, our attempts to love will always meet with a measure of frustration. And yet, we continue to seek this total identity with the other, to give ourselves totally and lose ourselves in the person of our beloved. And to the degree to which we are able to do so, we share in the beauty of the Divine love.

It was by total love, the complete giving of self, that Christ redeemed us. When He came to His people, He came as a bridegroom. When asked why His disciples did not fast, He answered: *"Can the wedding guests fast as long as the bridegroom is with them? As long as they have the bridegroom with them they cannot fast. But the days will come when the bridegroom shall be taken away from them, and then they will fast on that day* (Mk. 2 : 18–21). Claiming the identity of the bridegroom, and speaking of his disciples as the bridegroom's friends, Christ was clearly telling His listeners that He was, indeed, the Messiah they had been promised.

Identifying Himself as the bridegroom, Christ fulfilled the prophecies and also revealed what was to be His relationship with His Church. The Church was to be His bride. It was to be a union of love, a seeking to become one. As the perfect bridegroom, His love was sacrificial; willingly, he "delivered himself up" for His bride. As His bride, the Church can seek no identity apart from His. It is a total submission, in love, to Him.

Repeatedly, we find marriage used as the symbol of this union (Matt. 9 : 15; 25 : 1–13; John 3 : 29; 2 Cor. 11 : 2; Eph. 5 : 23–32; Apoc. 19 : 7–9; 21 : 9). In pondering the words of Christ and His apostles, the Church, during the first centuries, was able to recognize its identity as His bride and, at the same time, discover the significance of this revelation to the sacrament of Matrimony. In his fifth letter to the Christians of the City of Ephesus, St. Paul presented the ideal of the sacrament and the role of the spouses in the redeemed state as well as a metaphorical description of Christ's union with His Church. This epistle, read during the nuptial mass, answers the question, "Why was marriage raised to the new, and higher, dignity of a sacrament?"

Be subject to one another in the fear of Christ. Let wives be subject to their husbands as to the Lord; because a husband is head of the wife, just as Christ is head of the Church, being himself savior of the body. But just as the Church is subject to Christ, so also let wives be to their husbands in all things.

Husbands, love your wives, just as Christ also loved the Church, and delivered Himself up for her, that He might sanctify her, cleansing her in the bath of water by means of the word; in order that He might present to Himself the Church in all her glory, not having spot or wrinkle or any such thing, but that she might be holy and without blemish. Even thus ought husbands also to love their wives as their own bodies. He who loves his own wife, loves himself. For no one ever hated his own flesh; on the contrary he nourishes and cherishes it, as Christ also does the Church (because we are members of his body, made from his flesh and from his bones). For this cause a man shall leave his father and mother and cleave to his wife; and the two shall become one flesh. This is a great mystery—I mean in reference to Christ and to the Church. However, let each one of you also love his wife just as he loves himself; and let the wife respect her husband (Eph. 5:21-33).

Thus, marriage was to become a "life in Christ," the

sacramental life to which we are called in Baptism. It was
not raised to a sacrament in order to make it holy; it had
been holy from the very beginning. Like all sacraments,
it is to fulfill a function, to play a very special role, in the
continuation of the redemptive act. Those called to this
vocation are to bring the world to Christ, and to witness
Christ to the world, through their vocation; living their
marriage, they are to "show forth Christ."

The sexual love of the Christian husband and wife has
not, however, always been viewed as a witnessing sign of
Christ. In the Judaic culture of the early Church, the
words of St. Paul must have struck a strange chord indeed.
After all, wives had not been accorded this dignity since
Eden. Now, no longer were they to be slaves. Now, liber-
ated, they could give themselves freely to their husbands.
The marital union was again to be one of love, the love
of two equals, in which man and woman fulfill their complementary roles, neither exploiting nor being exploited.
But this was a far cry from the realities of that time, and it
was an ideal which few could grasp and even fewer could
accept. The change would come slowly. Much of the early
writing on sexuality and marriage, therefore, even by the
most esteemed Fathers of the Church, seems strangely at
variance with the ideal. Some is blatantly anti-sexual, anti-
feminine, and only tolerant of marriage. There were re-
curring heresies suggesting that the sexual union, even
within Christian marriage, was evil. Very few voices
spoke of its beauty and sacredness. True, the heresies were
successfully combated and the Church at no time questioned the licitness of marital sexuality, but a cloud remained, and throughout the early Church little was written
of love in the sacrament of Matrimony.

In part, the negativism toward marriage and the anti-
sexualism so prominent in the writings of many centuries,
reflected cultural values resistant to change. The ideal set

forth so beautifully by St. Paul, however, remained, and we can feel quite sure that there were many couples, much like Priscilla and Aquila (Acts 18 : 26), living the beauty and holiness of their union. But these were voices which were seldom heard. Hence, Christian marriage became the "silent vocation."

Marital sexuality, in particular, seemed strangely removed from the Life in Christ to which husband and wife were called. Too often discussed only within the context of moral theology and canon law, love again seemed, if not lost, at least misplaced. Philosophers sought to analyze the *purpose* of sexuality, but seldom its *meaning*. This frequently led to an emphasis on the procreative function to the neglect of conjugal *love*. And this, in turn, resulted in accusations that the Church viewed marriage solely in terms of procreation. We need not attempt to trace the source of the one-sided biologism which marked some of this writing; it is enough to admit, sorrowfully, that it was written, and to recognize, regretfully, that it still exists in the scrupulous thinking of some Christian couples.

Nevertheless, the ideal of Eden has never been abandoned. Time and again the Church, speaking with the voice of Christ, has spoken the words of the gospels—"THAT TWO SHALL BECOME ONE" (Matt. 19 : 5). She has repeatedly defended the sanctity and beauty of sexual love in the vocation of Christian marriage, combating the forces of secularization and amorality which would strip marriage and conjugal love of the dignity established by the God "Who made man from the beginning male and female" (Matt. 19 : 4). Once more, the Church spoke out at Vatican II to "offer guidance and support to those Christians and other men who are trying to preserve the holiness and to foster the natural dignity of the married state and its superlative value."

"Christ the Lord abundantly blessed this many-faceted

love, welling up as it does from the fountain of divine love and structured as it is on the model of His union with His Church. For as God of old made Himself present to His people through a covenant of love and fidelity, so now the Savior of men and the Spouse of the Church comes into the lives of married Christians through the sacrament of Matrimony. He abides with them thereafter so that just as He loved the Church and handed Himself over on her behalf, the spouses may love each other with perpetual fidelity through mutual self-bestowal."

In an age in which *sexuality* is thought by many to be virtually synonymous with *immorality*, the Fathers of the Council forthrightly spoke out for the "right ordering" of sexual love and the purity and holiness of the marital union. There was no "puritanism" or Jansenism in their words, only the ideal of love and the message of the gospels telling of Christ's redeeming power enriching and strengthening this sublime gift of self.

"This love is an eminently human one since it is directed from one person to another through an affection of the will; it involves the good of the whole person, and therefore can enrich the expressions of body and mind with a unique dignity, ennobling these expressions as special ingredients and signs of the friendship distinctive of marriage. This love God has judged worthy of special gifts, healing, perfecting and exalting gifts of grace and of charity. Such love, merging the human with the divine, leads the spouses to a free and mutual gift of themselves, a gift providing itself by gentle affection and by deed; such love pervades the whole of their lives: indeed by its busy generosity it grows better and grows greater. Therefore it far excels mere erotic inclination, which, selfishly pursued, soon enough fades wretchedly away."

The return to Eden is painfully slow. At one time the path may seem clearer than at another, and less strewn with obstacles, but at best, it is always uphill and we see the way only "through a glass darkly." Hence, we stumble many times. We know the difficulties and the failures encountered along the way. We, too, are walking this road and climbing this mountain. So in speaking of the ideal we don't intend to deny the obvious. It is an ideal. And an ideal is never humanly attainable; if we can reach it, it is less than an ideal; our sights are set too low. Conjugal love, like all human love, must be placed at the service of values which are transcendent. If not, the marital relationship will become all too "human," with all the "human" problems, "human" solutions (and lack of them), "human" frustrations, and "human" despair. Christian marriage can never be simply a natural state; it must be stamped with the supernatural or it will fail. The path toward Eden is the path toward union in God through our deepening participation in the Redemption. Our progress will be measured by our growth in the mystery of love, that love "which the Lord revealed to the world by His dying and His rising up to life again."

The union in love of our first parents is the promise, a union in the Life of Christ. Our goal can be nothing less. Can we dream of anything more? A lifelong honeymoon, one planned by God.

CHAPTER II

Sexual Attitudes

RECENTLY, WE participated in a panel discussion of "Sex Education of the Pre-teen-age Child." The five panelists were all experienced professional workers in the area of parent-child relationships. Unfortunately, we had no time before the program in which to compare notes, and as we each, in turn, presented short preliminary papers, we became embarrassingly aware that we were all saying essentially the same thing. During the question period which followed, it also became evident that many in the audience felt frustrated and disappointed. They had come for specific answers and were given none. They had expected to hear opinions on how a child should be given the "facts of life," what "facts" should be given, when, and by whom. Instead, the panelists all said, in effect, "These are not the important issues." The so-called "facts of life," that is, the elementary anatomy and physiology of reproduction, can be picked up in a fifteen- or twenty-minute reading of a pamphlet. What is most important is the formation of sexual *attitudes,* and this is seldom the product of a book or pamphlet—or even a carefully worded lecture on the birds and bees. Nor does this formation of attitudes start with adolescence or the pre-teens, or even the first time the child asks the question, "Where did I come from?" We might say that the child's sexual attitudes germinate before the child is weaned from its bottle. The reaction of the parents to two-year-old Johnny parading downstairs naked, the way mother handles the incident of five-year-old Mary playing "doctor" with her friends, the physical affection the child sees expressed between his parents, these lay the foundation for the formation of sexual attitudes, attitudes which will then be carried through childhood and ado-lescence and, ultimately, into marriage—for better or for worse.

Often couples will ask, "How do we teach our children proper attitudes toward sex?" There is no simple answer to this question, no clear guidelines. The final answer can only be, "Look to yourselves; examine your values and attitudes." The best assurance we have of our children developing healthy and holy attitudes toward sexuality is to develop such attitudes in ourselves. The sexually frigid wife who told us she saw no reason to do anything about the problem is sadly mistaken. She is tragically in error in assuming that her daughter, having merely been told that "sex is good," will mature with healthy sexual attitudes. The "messages" we communicate to a child are more frequently non-verbal. And the child can be expected to have incorporated many of the parental attitudes long before he or she is conscious of any strictly sexual thoughts and feelings. These learned emotional reactions may be unverbalized and largely un-conscious, but they are often deeply rooted and, therefore, not easily unlearned. Nor can they usually be dispelled by simple instruction. The child, for instance, may be told that the body is to be revered as the temple of the Holy Spirit but, no matter how often he may hear the words, they will probably have little meaning for him if his mother holds the feelings expressed by one wife: "I find my husband's body very attractive—from the waist up!"

An individual's attitudes toward sexuality can seldom be

described as simply "good" or "bad," "healthy" or "un-healthy." They can probably best be thought of as on a continuum. Perhaps none of us possess perfect "health" in our attitudes, and, fortunately, relatively few can be described as seriously "ill." We might say that the degree to which our sexual attitudes contribute to the attainment of the total *oneness* which is Christian marriage, is the degree to which they can be considered "healthy," and, conversely, the degree to which they act to deter us in this quest, will be the measure of their "unhealthiness." The test, then, is whether our attitudes, and the behavior which is reflective of them, aid that mutual growth in Christ which is the challenge of our vocation.

Unfortunately, as we look about, there often seem to be more negative than positive forces operating to influence our sexual attitudes. Worse yet, it isn't always easy to perceive such negative influences. At times they seem to be functioning at a subliminal level. A television play or novel glorifying adultery can at least be seen for what it is: pathetic, or evil, or both. But where the influence is less obvious, where, in fact, it may masquerade as good, identifying it as evil may be difficult. Rooting out the resultant attitudes may be even more difficult.

In attitude formation, words are very important. A rose by any other name may indeed still be a rose, but attitudes are shaped by the words we choose. Sexual attitudes, perhaps more than all others, are revealed by our choice of words, the labels we attach to things sexual. We speak of "dirty" jokes and "dirty" stories. But is there anything dirty in human sexuality? Certainly, these jokes and stories often present sex in an irreverent manner. Frequently they have as their theme adultery, fornication, or even perversion. But what is it that we call *dirty?* So many of the words we employ communicate the same attitude: *smutty, filthy, off-color.* In defending the use of these words, the explanation usually offered is that it is not sexuality, per se, but immoral sexual behavior which is "dirty." We may be thinking of some metaphorical "stain on the soul." But if so, then surely stealing, slander, and murder are at least as "dirty." Why is it only sexual immorality which is "dirty"?

One wife in her mid-thirties, married ten years, had never permitted her husband to see her undressed. Her explanation was that she would not want to do anything which might give her husband *impure* thoughts! It became apparent through our discussions that both she and her husband equated *purity* with non-sexual, and *impurity* with anything sexual. As we might expect, they both found marital relations less than satisfying. Sexual love can never grow into *love* so long as it is viewed as impure. Unfortunately, we cannot cite this couple as an exceptional case; they have much company; their attitudes are only, perhaps, an extreme example. The sheer number of such cases makes it more than a tragedy. Their attitudes are distorted; the concepts of purity and impurity are confused; but in the way in which these concepts were presented in their childhood, such confusion is inevitable.

Like so many children, they were instructed in purity at an age when it could be nothing more than a meaningless word, a vague abstraction. Even if it could have had meaning for a child, the concept was never really defined. Little was actually communicated except the undefined words, *purity* and *impurity*. They were told to shun "impure thoughts and actions," to strive for "purity in mind and body." But what were the "impure thoughts" they were to avoid? This was never explained. But could it have been? So that it was understandable to a child? Probably not. Instead, all they learned was that there is some sort of dreadful sin associated with some sort of dreadful thoughts. A priest friend of ours talked of the eight- and nine-year-olds confessing to the "sin" of adultery. We may, at first, find amusement in the story, but when we stop to consider its implications, the humor vanishes. The child has been taught that adultery is a mortal sin. Whatever the act "committed," the child believes it to be adultery. (Another priest told of questioning a child about such confessed "adultery" and discovering that the boy had sinned by urinating in the bushes.) Furthermore, most of these children can give a very graphic description of the fiery hell awaiting those who die in mortal sin. There is little humor in the fear that these thoughts can arouse in the child.

All sorts of thoughts and actions may come to be labeled *impure* by the child. A second-grader may believe that kissing his younger sister is sinful. A nine-year-old girl may feel that viewing her baby brother fresh from his morning bath is wrong or "nasty." The words *purity* and *impurity*, along with the other words frequently used in reference to sexuality, often lead to an association developing between sexuality and cleanliness, and even bodily functions. One priest has called this the "Ivory soap concept" of sexuality. The child hears mother remark that the baby is "dirty" and in need of a change of diapers; but mother may also attempt to discourage the child from handling its genitals by employing the same word: "Mustn't touch yourself there; it's dirty." The one becomes associated with the other and the child learns to view the genital organs as dirty or ugly. Consciously or unconsciously, many carry this association into marriage.

Similar confused "messages" often mark the teaching of modesty. We tell a child that modesty is a virtue, but too often it is not a virtue we are teaching—or that we were taught. Again, the virtue is seldom defined. Instead, certain dress and behavior are pointed out and labeled "immodest"; other actions and dress are described as "modest." From this, the child is presumably to draw some generalization, some over-all rules governing dress and behavior. But how realistic is this expectation? The distinctions and discriminations demanded often make very little sense to an adult—to say nothing of a child. Modesty is always relative. The distinctions must be drawn within the framework of a host of environmental conditions. What may be modest at one time and place would be immodest at another. The native girl, nude to the waist, kneeling to receive the Blessed Sacrament on a South Pacific atoll, cannot be censured for immodesty. And yet, we don't teach this. Too often, modest and immodest dress and behavior, and the criteria which are to govern them, are taught as if they were absolutes, and not dependent upon age, time, place, and circumstance.

Many husbands and wives enter marriage with unhealthy attitudes stemming from this absolutist approach. More are merely confused and uncertain. They may believe that there are some "rules" of modesty which apply in the relationship of husband and wife; they are not so sure, however, what such limits may be. This would not present a major problem if the solution could be found in properly instructing the couple in a different set of "rules," one more suitable to marriage. Unfortunately, this seldom is very effective. Our attitudes are not held on a purely cognitive or rational level. They are, to a great extent, emotional, learned early, and usually reinforced over many years. They may be irrational, but they are not easily changed. Modesty and immodesty are taught with an association of shame, and the concepts cannot be given by teaching shame without the concepts becoming submerged and only a revulsion for the body remaining. We may tell a couple that their notion of modesty (implicitly defined as a hiding of the body) has no place in the intimacy of marriage, but if the young bride has been taught that the female breasts should not only be covered but concealed, she may not be able to walk, nude, to meet her husband's embrace without experiencing embarrassment, shame, or even guilt. She may feel that the filmy negligee he gives to her is somehow improper, that his suggestion that they shower together is degrading. The fears and inhibitions she brings to marriage may thus cause her to set limits and restrict the freedom of emotional expression necessary for their growth in love.

Even if the couple are able to cast off these inhibitions and discover the excitement to be found in an open physical expression of their love, a residual of these unhealthy attitudes may remain and deprive their sexual love of its intended fulfillment. In finding the pleasure derived from a complete physical acceptance of each other, they may even, ironically, lose the oneness that could, and should, be the goal of marriage. Sexuality, although pleasurable, may be felt to be somehow illicit. Hence, in its attraction, it will carry the scent of "forbidden fruit." Consequently, their sexual love will not become integrated into the *whole* marriage. It will remain compartmentalized and divorced from their spiritual relationship, as if their sexual relations will profane, rather than bless, their sacramental vocation.

If there is, in fact, any core problem, it is this compartmentalization of sexuality. Nearly all books on marriage attempt to answer the questions of what *part* sex plays in marriage, and what part it should play. But these questions imply that sexuality can be quantified. Is it twenty per cent or eighty per cent? Of course, probably none of these writers intend to treat marital sexuality as if it were a matter of percentages, but their implication, unfortunately, is that it is merely one activity, of many, in the marriage. The same attitude is reflected when we speak of the *sex life* of a husband and wife—as if it were split off from the remainder of the couple's existence.

Viewed as it should be, sexuality is not some *part* of

marriage. It is the *total* marriage! Everything in the relationship between husband and wife is sexual—in the broadest and deepest meaning of the word. It is the relationship between a man and a woman, two individuals of complementary sex joined in an inseparable and mysterious union. Everything in their relationship reflects their sexual identities. From the cup of coffee she pours for him in the morning until they fall asleep in each other's arms, they emotionally interact, not merely as two human beings, but as a man to a woman and a woman to a man. Where the couple have attained that unity which should be the goal of those called to the vocation of Christian marriage, it is no more realistic to think and speak of a "sex life" than of a "dishwashing life," an "eating life," or even a "prayer life." They have one life, one marriage, one quest for fulfillment and salvation. Theirs is a single identity which they strive to perfect. In the physical expression of their love, their separate and distinct sexual identities merge, synthesize, and grow in a oneness which symbolizes their sacramental vocation.

In order for the personalities of the couple to fuse in this manner, the attitudes of both husband and wife toward their own sexuality and sexual identity must be wholesome. The husband must know what he is *as a man*, and the wife must know what she is *as a woman*. If there is any single *sine qua non* of a successful marriage, it is that a *man* marry a *woman*, and vice versa. Unfortunately, not all adult males who enter marriage are *men*, and many of the wives are not *women*.

As human beings, our primary identity is that of our sex. We are born male or female; we become men or women. But what is a man and what is a woman? In spite of (or because of?) a plethora of recent books and essays discussing, debating, and dissecting the nature and roles of the contemporary male and female, most husbands and wives are hopelessly confused as to what they are as well as what they are intended to be. They have little understanding of their own sexual nature and even less understanding of the sexual nature of the one to whom they are married. Often, they are unsure of what attitudes they should or should not hold, what feelings they should or should not have, what desires are "normal" or not for a man or for a woman. Again and again we hear the question, "Is it normal for a woman (or a man) to feel such-and-such?"

Unless a woman is secure and unself-conscious in what she feels, and is fully aware and sure of her womanhood, and unless her husband is certain and secure in his manhood, their sexual relations will suffer. Just as sexuality is not some part, only, of marriage, it is not merely some *part* of the human personality. It reflects the entire personality. In marriage, the couple attempt to merge their complementary personalities. And in the sexual union, the total personalities of each are revealed to the other. Such total exposure of self, however, can be threatening, and even painful. Hence, if the couple are confused, anxious, or ashamed of their sexual feelings, they will hold back, fearful of such exposure. The openness and freedom in communication necessary to the development of physical love will be absent; consequently, sexual relations will serve, at most, to satisfy merely a physical drive.

For the marriage to grow, both must be able to find the spiritual meaning in marital relations, to see the image of their Creator in the human body (all the body—not excluding the genital organs), and to accept, gratefully, the strength of their sexual desires. The development will be slow and painful, however, if they have been taught to view all sexual urges as temptations and sexual arousal as sinful. They will have much to overcome. Nevertheless, unhealthy sexual attitudes can be overcome, and positive attitudes developed. And they must if the marriage is to reach fulfillment. The motivation necessary to make the effort should stem, at least in part, from a recognition that healthy sexual attitudes are essential to the total growth of the marriage.

Many wives have been taught a distorted concept of the sexual nature of a woman. They have been told that a woman "by nature" has less sexual drive than a man, that she is less passionate, less frequently and intensely aroused, and even that strong sexual desire—and satisfaction—is not a part of her nature. Despite a sizable body of evidence to the contrary, there are still some popular writers (albeit, poorly informed) who contend that women are essentially asexual. One such writer, a syndicated columnist, virtually implied that it is normal for women to be frigid. "Most wives," he claimed, "are satisfied with nothing more than a good night kiss."

It should come as no surprise to find this notion still prevalent. Old myths and fallacies die hard and seem easily resurrected. And this one has been with us a long time. Too long. It has been only since the turn of the century that serious attempts have been made to systematically study human sexuality. Before, what writing there was on the subject was based more on mores and censures (what the writer felt should be true) than on empirical findings. A distinguished physician living in Victorian England, for example, was reflecting nothing other than the culture in which he lived when he denounced as "despicable" and "slanderous" the suggestion that a "lady" might experience erotic feelings. Even the eminent pioneer sexologist, Richard von Krafft-Ebing (1840–1902), asserted that, "Since woman has less sexual need than man, a predominating sexual desire in her arouses a suspicion of its pathological significance." Although Krafft-Ebing was writing here of what he termed *hyperaesthesia*, an abnormal increase in sexual desire, it is significant that he views that which might be considered normal in a man as symptomatic of pathology in a woman!

In many respects we may be far removed from the culture of Victorian England. Most certainly, our contemporary society cannot be accused of any puritanical suppression of sex. And yet, we still see wives who seem convinced that any admission of sexual pleasure is a mark of wantonness. The result is sad indeed. For them, sexual relations remain at the level of a "masculine prerogative." And so long as they expect nothing more, they don't seek it. Their mistaken belief that women are essentially asexual, or at least that they have a much lower sexual drive than their husbands, cripples them and their marriage, although often without their being aware of it. And little wonder, in view of the support given such beliefs. How many times, for example have these wives listened to the wife's role in marital relations described as the "wifely duty"? How many times have they heard talk of the husband's "marital rights"? Shades of a female martyr chained to the stake!

Certainly men and women differ in their sexual response, just as they differ in anatomy and physiology. Man and woman are, after all, of different sex. These differences, in a good marriage, result in a wonderful interaction. Partly, this is what is meant when we speak of the sexes as *complementary*. Through the expression of their sexuality, these very different human beings blend in such a beautiful way that to ponder it is to come to the realization that these very differences are one of God's choicest gifts. What glory was given to Him by the elderly French politician who cried out, "*Vive la différence!*"

The difference in sexual response, however, is *qualitative*, not *quantitative*. We can't measure its strength and make comparisons. It makes as little sense to talk of the sexual response of one sex as more intense or pleasurable as it would to argue that a painting by Raphael is more aesthetic than a symphony by Beethoven. The pleasure and satisfaction experienced by a normal woman, while different from that of her husband, is at least as deep and profound. And her sex drive is as strong. If, in fact, we could compare the magnitude of response, there are a number of reasons why we might expect to find her drive stronger, and her satisfaction greater!

For one thing, woman is far more complex sexually. Her sexuality extends to every part of her being. While its physiology is still not fully known, the affect of her sexuality on her total make-up, both physical and psychological, can hardly be overestimated; in contrast, the sexual physiology of man seems almost elementary.

But women, unfortunately, are taught to stifle their sexual feelings, and to accept the fallacy that they were created with a "normal" attitude of sexual indifference. Hence, as we might expect, what we frequently see in wives is a rather pathetic conflict. If love and affection grow in the marriage, as they should, the wife can expect to experience increased sexual desire and deeper sexual satisfaction. Through her marriage, she grows into womanhood; and this, in part, is expressed through her sexual feelings. But if she has been taught to view these feelings as "unnatural"—that is, not in keeping with the nature of woman—she will find herself caught in a painful paradox: as she becomes *more* a woman, she begins to fear that she is *less* than womanly. Reacting to this fear, she may attempt to suppress her feelings and/or conceal them from her husband.

To add to the problem, the conflict she feels may be intensified by her husband. If he, too, has been raised in sexual ignorance and believes women have less sexual desire and are "satisfied with nothing more than a good night kiss," he may approach marital relations as his "marital right" and nothing more. He may be unaware of any obligation to make *love* to his wife. But while his interests may extend no further than satisfaction of his own desires, we can't say that his actions are necessarily callous and unloving. After all, if women are really as sexually insensitive as he believes, making love would be a wasted effort!

We have listened to wives, caught in this dilemma, apprehensively admit to feelings of strong sexual desire as if they were confessing to a perversion. Some have expressed them to their husbands only to find their spouses were repulsed by such "unwomanly" emotions. One such husband actually sought psychotherapy for his wife. He felt sure her open expression of sexual desire was a sign of emotional illness!

If there is another side to this coin, it is the equally destructive notion that men "by nature" are driven by a strong biological force which *demands* an outlet—almost any outlet. The protagonists of this view argue that men are innately predatory and polygamous. And in the end, they reduce sexual relations to mere physical actions, wholly devoid of psychological or spiritual meaning. This concept of manhood is stated, implied, restated, and reinforced in men's magazines, motion pictures, television plays, and marriage manuals. Even some Christian writers are not immune. After repeating the fallacy, one such writer concluded: "For this reason, it is possible for a man to have sexual intercourse with a woman other than his wife without ceasing to love his wife." (We can only wonder how this writer defines "love"!)

Raised under a continual bombardment of this influence, many husbands adopt the role they have been told is "natural." They attempt to project this "masculine" image: the philandering playboy, scoring sexual conquests, living in a "he-man" world of mental (if not physical) adultery, sexually exploiting but seldom loving. To admit deeper emotions, or to express tenderness and love, would threaten the image. In attempting to polish his virile image, one playboy husband flippantly remarked: "Making love has no more meaning than taking a drink of water; it relieves your thirst and it's pleasant, but why try to make anything more of it?" The "why" we might ask in answer is, "Why, if it has no more meaning than you say, do you call it 'making love'?" Certainly, the meaning in sexual relations may not be clear to the particular couple, although it should be. And what is communicated may even be unhealthy and unloving. But *every* act in sexual relations communicates some meaning. To suppress or deny meaning, is to take from the act that which makes it human. It depersonalizes it. And it depersonalizes the total relationship.

Many wives have also been taught this erroneous concept of the masculine "nature." Throughout childhood, they may have listened to the words: "All men are . . ." from the lips of embittered mothers. The result: They expect their husbands to be adulterous—at least in thought if not in behavior. They believe what they have been told: "Men are interested in only one thing."

In clinging to these misconceptions, both husband and wife interact by role-playing, each acting out a distorted stereotype of their sex. Communication never develops in their sexual relations—or in any area. The conjugal union is merely an *act*, nothing more. And they become little more than automatons, devoid of feeling, routinely fulfilling a marital obligation.

But even here they fail. The obligations of marriage can never be met by the mere performance of an act or the mere giving of a service. They can only be fulfilled through loving. And love, sexual or otherwise, is the giving of *self*, not the giving of service. There are, to be sure, serious sexual obligations in marriage, but they extend far beyond what is implied by any "services rendered."

We said the obligation is to *love*. In the sexual embrace, this is expressed by attempting to *fully* meet the needs and desires of the other; that is, by continually striving to increase the other's enjoyment and satisfaction. This is the giving of self; and it is this giving which transforms the sexual *act* into sexual *love*. The actions of each are motivated by the desires of the other. Both look to the other, searching for the frequently subtle cues that point to the ways of loving. Each strives to "hear" the other, to recognize, in the actions of love, the ever-changing needs, hopes, desires, and fears revealed.

For this loving to develop, preconceived concepts which tend to stereotype the sexes must be recognized as destructive, and a constant effort must be made to *see* the other as he or she really *is*. This is seldom easy; it is usually much less effort to fall back on the sexual stereotypes we have learned. Often, the explanation we give ourselves for the behavior, needs, and desires of our spouse is really no explanation at all. We merely dismiss their words and actions with the statement, "That's the way he (or she) is." This is somewhat like the answer a child gives when asked: "Why?" "Just *because*, that's why."

As in psychotherapy, where the therapist must listen "with the third ear," striving to understand what the patient is "saying" beneath the surface words, husband and wife must seek to discover the underlying motivations and needs of the other. But in order for the psychotherapist to be able to effectively "listen," he must know himself and the blind spots in his own personality which might stand in the way of his helping others. Similarly, husband and wife must probe their own personalities and know themselves so that they may know each other. They must examine their feelings and attitudes and attempt to rid themselves of any unhealthy sexual attitudes and emotional reactions which tend to inhibit the complete giving of self. With most, this will mean a rather thorough "self-analysis"; with others, where a deeper problem exists, professional counseling may be indicated.

The importance of developing healthy and holy attitudes toward sexuality is brought into focus when we consider the extent of our marital obligations. Sexual love, even in its most loving sense, will be incomplete unless both find satisfaction and fulfillment. In addition to striving to give satisfaction to one's spouse, there is a positive duty to seek to increase one's own sexual pleasure. We cannot, of course, say that the wife whose only satisfaction in marital relations is the pleasure she gives to her husband is not loving. Certainly she is. She is giving of herself, and this, by definition, is loving. But the meaning and growth of Christian marriage is bound to the meaning and growth of the marital union. It is complex and all-inclusive; and the multiple purposes served by sexual love in a Christian marriage cannot be met by such unilateral giving of self.

Thus, our obligation is twofold; to give sexual fulfillment, and to strive to achieve it. In subsequent chapters we will examine the physical, psychological, and spiritual dimensions of marital sexuality. An understanding of this dual obligation rests on an understanding of each of these, and of the ways in which they interact. And above all, it rests on an understanding of love.

CHAPTER III

The Husband

WHEN A BRIDE takes "this man," she makes a commitment *to* him as a person, and *with* him to a life of Christian perfection. It is a commitment made with trust that through him she will find fulfillment as a woman. Hence, it is made with confidence in him *as a man*.

She may not be able to clearly describe her image of manhood. It may be vague or unrealistic. It may even be an expression of her own neurotic needs. But in any case, she will have some sort of image. Long before she meets the man she will marry, this image will have been formed. And once formed, all men will be evaluated against the criteria of this image.

In the last chapter, we spoke of the increasing confusion of sex roles. We see its effect in numerous ways and in scores of marriages. But the image the wife holds is not confused. She knows, or at least thinks she knows, what she is seeking. And so, verbalized in a variety of expressions, one of the most frequent complaints heard in psychotherapy with couples is that of the wife: "I wish my husband were a *man!*"

The accusation is more than serious. It penetrates to the foundation of the relationship. Unless she is able to see him as a *man*, and unless he is able to feel secure in his manhood, every aspect of their marriage will be adversely affected. Since sexuality, both in a general and specific sense, rests on sexual identity, their marital relations will most surely be less than fully satisfactory.

Much has been written of the prevalence of non-men. It is not a new social problem by any means. Apparently, however, it is growing at a frightening rate. There seem to be fewer and fewer *men,* and their absence increasingly affects the social structure. The solution is as elusive as the problem is complex. When we attempt to analyze it, we find ourselves caught in many "chicken or the egg" dilemmas. Are more women, for example, becoming masculine "of necessity" because they are married to non-men, or are husbands being emasculated in greater numbers by their wives? Or is it that the identities of both are being lost, and hence more non-men tend to marry more non-women?

Whatever the cause, these are invariably pathetic marriages. Both spouses have neurotic needs, and they seek satisfaction of them through the marriage, to the ultimate misery of both. They may even, in fact, receive a satisfaction of sorts, but nevertheless, it is a destructive interaction; to the extent such a symbiotic relationship is neurotic, it will result in unhappiness. Take, for example, a woman with a strong desire to dominate. She may marry a passive, dependent man, and in doing so meet her neurotic need. But in time, the roles they play can be counted on to frustrate both of them and erode their marriage. In one such case, the wife complained that her husband expected her to handle all of the family finances. She figured the budget, paid the bills, and decided on nearly all purchases, all of which she bitterly resented. And yet, even during their engagement period she had managed all of the money for both of them, even the disposition of his weekly pay check—a task she had taken over from his mother!

Non-men and non-women often come from similar environments. The homes from which they come may appear to be very different, but the same destructive elements are present in each. They are homes which lack any clear structuring of the parental roles. Often, they are homes in which the father is absent or, even if he is physically present, assumes little of the responsibility of fatherhood in rearing the children. Hence, the children are raised almost entirely by their mother. There is no chance for the sons to identify with their father, nor for the girls to learn something of the appropriate roles of the sexes in marriage. As a result, there is very little development of a mature sexual identity. These homes are not the exception, unfortunately. They may even constitute the majority. Time and again, we see husbands, raised in such homes, who are as confused about what it is to be a *man* as their wives are embittered at not having married one.

To understand the frustration of such a wife and what she is seeking in her husband, we might start by describing what she does *not* mean when she speaks of a *man*. First of all, she is not longing for the hypervirility of an Ernest Hemingway hero. Manhood, to her, will not be proven through big-game hunting, armed combat, or sexual conquests. These may form a caricature of masculinity, but what she wants is a man, not a caricature.

This is a part of the problem, however. The caricature has almost become the norm. Our society, with *men*—real *men*—in the minority, has produced an image of masculinity which is a contradiction, one which is antithetical to manhood. The image is narrow, two-dimensional, and distorted. It presents manhood stripped of all nobility, all sensitivity. And all humanity.

And so many non-men accept it. Plagued by fears that others may perceive in them a lack of masculinity, many husbands attempt to project this image. They shun all behavior which they see as indicative of a deficiency in manliness. But in order to accomplish this, they dichotomize the sexes in a wholly unrealistic manner: they class nearly all interests and attitudes as "masculine" or "feminine." The emphasis—and over-emphasis—is on the sexes as *opposite* rather than complementary. All "feminine" interests are suppressed and ridiculed. These usually include the aesthetic and all interests, actions, and reactions which might be considered romantic, emotional, or spiritual. Thus, art, poetry, romantic love, and religion are viewed by the hypervirile husband as unmanly and he dares not be caught in anything unmanly.

The mass media do more than their share to foster this. Take, for example, the heroes of television Westerns and war dramas. As boorish as they are, they present many a grown-up little boy with an opportunity to identify with a hypervirile hero in a vicarious fantasy which often takes on the characteristics of a Walter Mitty flight from reality. But the dream world is usually short-lived, and soon such husbands are again caught up in the doubts and anxieties which surround their self-image. They seldom are successful in convincing themselves that they are truly men; they succeed only in shutting their eyes to the problem.

There is always a circularity to a negative self-image. The individual who sees himself as inadequate is compelled to erect defenses since to feel inadequate is to feel vulnerable. But the building and maintaining of these emotional defenses forces him to act in ways which ultimately only increase his feelings of inadequacy. Thus, the he-man façade which such an inadequate husband employs works to impede his attainment of manhood. The façade becomes a wall which locks out others, including his wife, and locks him inside. He can't establish close personal relationships; he is incapable of experiencing mature emotion and unable to give love or accept it.

And now let's look at a *man*. When we attempt to describe such a husband, several words come to mind. Take the word *strength,* for example. Perhaps more than all others, it stands for manhood—at least to most women. It is the essential masculine characteristic, the basic attribute which permits a wife to rely on her husband, to place all her trust in him and derive her strength from him.

An attractive widow in her fifties told us what this had meant to her. "John was my security, not in the way a child clings to a parent, not out of a feeling that I couldn't cope with the world alone, but because of what he was and what I am, because I am a woman and I needed him as a man; and because he needed to have me need him this way. Even during the last two years, when John could no longer care for himself and I became the sole support of the family, my strength still came from him. He was in every respect a *man.*"

A young mother of five spoke of finding the same characteristic in her husband when she emphasized his convictions. "It's what he believes in, what he stands for. The first year of our marriage I'm afraid I pushed pretty hard. I wanted to be able to put my trust in him, but I was scared. You see, I had always been pretty self-reliant and I was frightened at the prospect of totally relying on someone else. So, you might say I was testing the limits. Once I discovered, however, that I could go just so far and no further, that he had convictions that were not going to be swayed, that he firmly believed in and lived by, then I knew I could relax and follow his lead."

Like these two women, probably all wives look for this strength in their husbands. A wife has a need to feel that her husband is a pillar she can lean upon. But it is not so much that she needs this *from* him; she wants to give this *to* him. Psychologists use the word *dominance* to describe this strength in a man. Such masculine dominance is the hallmark of manhood. This should not, however, be confused with the word *domineering*. They are in no way similar characteristics. In fact, the dominant husband and the domineering husband are, if anything, at opposite ends of a continuum. The latter is autocratic, demanding, and most often a petty tyrant. Frequently, we find him to be the hypermasculine male we described. Rather than giving strength to his wife, he forces her to develop her own strength sufficiently to compensate for his weakness. Repeatedly, he reveals his insecurity by making capricious demands and by a childish display of temper. While he fashions himself into a dictatorial nineteenth-century patriarch, his wife provides the stability, emotional support, and love in the family. And so, in a final irony, the home becomes dominated by the wife and pervaded by momism.

The dominant husband, on the other hand, is not threatened in his masculinity, nor is he insecure in his role as husband and father. He, therefore, feels no need to assert his authority at every turn. He can freely love others without fearing that they will take advantage of him. While he is interested in, and accepting of, the opinions of others, he doesn't permit them to become the directing force in his life. He has a mind of his own and he uses it. He is able to make decisions and hold values confidently in spite of criticism. He nevertheless doesn't feel compelled to defensively justify his views to outsiders; he is secure enough to not feel attacked by those who hold differing views. It is this inner security which allows him to disregard the pressures from other husbands to join in their adolescent tales of mental adultery, nights-out-with-the-boys, and "he-man" escapes from responsibility.

The Christian husband-as-man accepts, without reservation, his responsibilities. But more than that, he welcomes them, even seeks them. And while they are his constant concern, they seldom become a source of anxiety. Supported by a sure reliance on Divine Providence, he has both faith in his judgment and confidence in his abilities, but at the same time he is not unaware of his limitations.

Husbands, love your wives, just as Christ also loved the Church, and delivered himself up for her (Eph. 5 : 2). There it is, succinctly stated, the obligation of the Christian husband: *to love*. He meets this obligation, primarily, through assuming his responsibilities, the total dedication implied in "delivering himself up for her." Through accepting his responsibilities in love, he attains manhood. Thus, the word *responsibile* is another key word in the definition of a *man*.

We see many husbands, however, who are singularly unaware of the scope of these responsibilities. They may be aware, for example, of the obligation to provide materially for their families, but fail to see that this is an obligation which must be understood within the context of the *whole* vocation, that is, in relation to all other obligations of the head of a family. But what we see are scores of husbands who apparently view the breadwinning role as their sole responsibility. Too often, they employ their obligations as wage earners to excuse their neglect of the family. They may, in fact, work very hard to provide their families with "everything money can buy," but they fail to comprehend the simple truth that marriage and parenthood cannot be purchased at any price. And the price they demand of themselves and their families buys only bitterness and contempt. They frequently provide no leadership, only a pay check, and yet they take pride in being "good providers."

To be sure, the demands of providing a livelihood may be heavy. They may demand sacrifices on the part of the husband as well as other members of the family. Approached with maturity and understanding, however, these pressures will not breed conflict between the spouses; they will be viewed as opportunities for growth. The conflicts arise not from the demands of work, but from rationalized exaggeration of these demands, and from a misguided hierarchy of values which places career above family. They arise when a husband attempts to demonstrate to the world his masculine prowess by climbing the ladder of a corporate structure, striving for professional status, or building a financial empire, and from them attempting to convince himself and others that his efforts are on behalf of his family—or, in other words, that his ambitions are a proof of his responsibility and concern. Yet let such a husband ask his wife. Unless she is consumed with material desires, her answer will be that she wants a man who is committed to his family, not to material goals.

Obviously, no list can be compiled that will include all the responsibilities and obligations of the head of a family. They may vary with changing circumstances, and they will always vary somewhat from one family to another. The essential responsibilities of a husband and father, however, are the same for all; they differ only in their implementation.

As soon as we mention the *headship of the family*, however, we expect to encounter resistance from some wives. This feminine rejection of the traditional role of the head of the family usually stems, however, from a misunderstanding of the role. In most cases, it has been viewed as a rather arbitrary claim to a *right*—which it isn't. The headship is not defined in terms of authority; it is not the "right to make decisions." Rather, it is defined in the assumption of responsibility. Any decision making will only follow as a natural consequence of this assumption. Responsibility without authority or authority without responsibility violate justice. And it is this injustice which is condemned by those who reject the concept of the headship of the family. If, for example, the husband capriciously makes decisions regarding the children when he has previously assumed little responsibility for their guidance, his wife may be justified in the resentment she feels. Responsibility coupled with authority equal *accountability*. And it is this which is the essence of the headship of a family. The husband is *accountable*. The burden rests on his shoulders. He is accountable for the material welfare of his family, for their secular and religious education, for their social and spiritual guidance. To be sure, he may delegate some of the teaching function to schoolteachers, Confraternity of Christian Doctrine instructors, and scoutmasters, and, most certainly, his wife will play a major role in rearing the children. But he cannot delegate the responsibility. It remains his. It is his responsibility to foster the faith which provides meaning, the hope which provides courage, and the love which provides security. This is the headship which a woman seeks to find in her husband. And it is this headship, the gentle direction of Christ, not the tyranny of a dictator, that a *man* strives to give to his family.

This is a book on sexuality, however, and what, you may ask, has all this to do with sexuality?

We previously said that sexuality, in both a general and specific sense, rests on sexual identity. In later chapters, we hope to expand on this and to examine the psychological implications inherent in the marital union and what it communicates between a man and woman. For now, we will only reiterate some of the points we have touched upon, placing them within the context of the masculine role in sexual relations.

In the sexual union, he makes a promise. All the pledges the husband makes to his bride when he takes her as a wife are implicitly renewed in his sexual overtures. In giving her body to him, she must totally surrender herself—if she is to achieve sexual fulfillment. In accepting her body, he promises to cherish and protect her, and in doing so, he reassures her in the trust she places in him. If he is faltering in these promises, however, or insecure in his manhood, she will be unable to experience this necessary security, and unable to surrender in love to her husband.

This also demands another kind of sureness on his part. For him to guide her in sexual love, he must have confidence in his ability to do so. She can greatly aid him in developing this confidence by the encouragement that comes from her loving response, but he, too, has a responsibility. In order to free her to respond sexually, he must first free himself. Any rigidity on his part, or false inhibitions, will be communicated to her and will limit her ability to respond. Thus, we might say that sex education in the broadest meaning of the word is more imperative for the husband than the wife. His role is that of both a gentle leader and a loving teacher.

It is more than strictly sexual leadership, however. Again and again we have listened to wives complain of a lack of completeness they experience in the sexual union. In nearly every case, the wife has told of a lack of confidence in her husband. These women are not saying, "I *will not* give obedience to my husband"; they're saying, "I *cannot*: I can't rely upon him enough to be able to do so." In most of these cases, the wife could not possibly follow her husband's direction; little or no direction is given!

There we have the third word: *leadership*. To be a man, he must lead, not follow, his wife; he must provide the direction for his family. His wife may live fully in the present; this is her nature as a woman; but he must at all times be concerned, at least to some degree, with the future. Countless plans must be made for his family: next week, next year, ten years hence. He must even plan for the welfare of his family in the event of his death. The home he provides for them, the income necessary to support them, the eventual college education of his children, demands planning. To lead his family, he must be ahead—in the future—not following behind in the past, or living only in the present.

This concern with the future also makes spiritual leadership a very natural part of his manhood. The vocation of Christian marriage is a religious vocation, a very special calling to what should become a beautiful journey toward mutual sanctity, and it is his direction which provides the roadmap for this journey. As he accepts the priesthood of the head of a family, he leads his wife and children toward heaven. This, perhaps more than all else, gives her the security she needs. It frees her to accept her vocation, to accept him, and to accept his sexual leadership; it frees her to become fully a woman. And it permits both to see sexual love as Christian love.

The demands of manhood are great indeed, but the rewards are still greater, and well worth striving toward. Manhood is seldom, if ever, easily attained. It is never a mere matter of learning the appropriate masculine role. It is not simply *doing* something; it is *being* something. And this is a growth process—often a very painfully slow growth process. Clear recognition of the responsibilities of manhood is the first step—but only the first step. Accepting these responsibilities and all that they entail comes next, and this is an awesome challenge. It demands that he give 100 per cent of himself. Not 50 per cent, nor even 99. *One hundred per cent!* It is the challenge to the attainment of sainthood—and to the attainment of manhood—which, in the vocation of the Christian husband, amount to the same thing.

CHAPTER IV

The Wife

SINCE THE SEXES are bipolar, we might be able to comprehend the nature of woman through an understanding of the nature of man. And conversely, we might grasp the meaning of manhood through a study of womanhood since each reaches maturity and fulfillment in their sexual nature through the other. But it would be a wise man indeed who *could* claim a thorough understanding of either sex. And perhaps only a fool who *would* make such a claim. We each have a serious obligation, however, to seek to understand something of the nature of both sexes.

Today, women are trying to understand themselves and their nature and role far more than to understand men. This may be a good thing since if they are to be able to understand their spouses, and, through their husbands, find fulfillment, they must begin with some valid self-insight. For many wives, however, this search seems endless, and they seldom seem any closer to finding answers. The questions they ask themselves (as well as others) touch on home, family, career, outside interests, and, of course, marriage. But implicitly, they are all asking the same questions. They are the existential questions, the answers to which would provide meaning to their lives. What does it mean to be a woman? A wife? What does the word fulfillment, a word so many use but so few understand, mean in the life of a wife and mother? There are answers to these questions, but they often become buried in the sounds of many voices competing to redefine the role of "woman in the modern world."

From every direction, wives are given advice. Self-styled experts are all too eager to discuss, analyze, and dissect what women *are* and what they should *become*. And their number is legion, but their effect is pernicious. They are perhaps responsible for much of the confusion and frustration felt by so many women. What they tell her she is to become is very often internally inconsistent; it can lead only to conflict should she attempt it. They may tell her, for example, that marriage is her vocation, but then encourage her to seek fulfillment outside of her home. Or an article may coach her in techniques for entertaining her husband's business associates, while the following article may emphasize her primary responsibility to her children. Should any wife attempt to accept and implement all that she is told she must be, she may find herself living in a very schizophrenic world.

Christian wives have not escaped these influences. If anything, the conflicts are even greater since they take on another and more serious aspect. They become centered in what she sees as her Christian commitment: obligation to home vs. obligation to parish; the role of the Christian wife vs. the role of the Christian mother, etc. The conflict, then, becomes one in conscience. What is a *Christian* woman? A *Christian* wife? A *Christian* mother?

First, how has the Church viewed the role of the Christian wife? Saint Paul tells us, *Let wives be subject to their husband as to the Lord; because a husband is head of the wife, just as Christ is head of the Church, being himself savior of the body. But just as the Church is subject to*

Christ, so also let wives be to their husbands in all things
(Eph. 5 : 2).

Being "subject," as the dictionary defines it, means "owing obedience or allegiance to the power or dominion of another." In our twentieth-century Western culture, this has a loud anachronistic ring to it, a return to the serfdom of the middle ages or perhaps the obsequious servility of the pre-Westernized oriental wife. And needless to say, this is pretty distasteful medicine to be asked to swallow. After all, we are living in an age in which women are no longer viewed as chattels and counted among the property of the lord of the manor along with the indentured servants and the oxen. Women are now recognized as human beings, equal in status to men, representing, as Cardinal Suenens reminded the Council members at Vatican II, approximately one half of the human race. Women are now playing a major role in the majority of professions, in the arts and sciences, and in the Church. The goals of the feminine emancipators of a half-century ago have been reached and surpassed beyond their furthest expectations. Is the Church then today asking women to give up the dignity and recognition they have achieved and to return to a subservient role? Could it be that the Church (as some feminists claim) views women as little more than "baby machines" whose only function, and hence worth, is the bearing of young?

These questions are important, but there is a far more fundamental issue: Is the wife's role, as taught by St. Paul, compatible with the *nature* of woman? If not, wives might justifiably rebel against it. If, on the other hand, the role is in keeping with woman's nature, why are we hearing an increasing number of Christian wives openly critical of the Church's teachings on the obligations of husband and wife, their roles, and even the Pauline metaphor?

We may begin to find some answers if we consider what

we observe in so many marriages. Time and again, we have listened to couples argue about their respective rights. During the question period following talks on marriage we are asked to answer countless questions which begin "Don't you believe a wife is entitled to . . ." or, "Isn't it true that a husband has a right to . . ." The concern of these questions is with justice, and justice only. Furthermore, and not unexpectedly, it nearly always involves something the questioner feels is owing them, almost never what they believe they might owe. But even if the approach is not totally self-seeking, a marriage cannot be built solely, or even primarily, on justice. We can go even a step further: discussion of the respective rights of the spouses is foreign to a good marriage, for while the virtue of justice is inherent in love, a good marriage is built on love, not justice.

Hence, if a woman being "subject" to her husband is taken to mean that she has been *subjugated,* the role she is being asked to assume is wholly incompatible with her nature—and opposed to the nature of marriage. Obviously, this cannot be what the Church is asking of the wife. She is to be a wife, not a slave.

She shares with her husband the obligation to *love,* to give of herself in the ways in which he needs to have her give. The key to the answer is found in the word *give.* Being subject to him is the gift, not demanded, but freely bestowed, which the wife gives to her husband. She willingly places her complete trust in him and follows his lead. This is never extracted from her, at least not in what we might describe as a good marriage. She desires the leadership of her husband. And the lack of leadership that so many wives find in their husbands forms the basis of the complaint we spoke of in the previous chapter: "My husband isn't a man!"

Many times, in speaking to groups of women, we have

made the assertion that all wives would like to be able to give obedience to their husbands, that is, to follow the leadership of their husbands, but, unfortunately, many feel they cannot do so. The statement may, of course, be too sweeping a generalization; there are, no doubt, some dedicated feminists who resist giving anything to any member of the opposite sex, not excluding their spouses. We find it interesting, however, and perhaps significant, that we have not yet had the statement challenged.

Lack of dependable leadership by the husband is the excuse offered by many wives when they claim they cannot follow their husbands. Usually, the claim is valid, but only partly. Often, the question is not so much why the wife *cannot* give, but why she *will not* give. In the answer to this question, seldom a single nor simple answer, may be found many of the explanations for the frustration and misery of the contemporary wife. Furthermore, and more directly related to our topic, it goes straight to the core of feminine sexuality and the disappointment so many women experience in the marital union.

Frigidity, the inability to achieve complete sexual satisfaction in intercourse, is so prevalent that some have come to accept it as "normal" (which, at least to some extent, may account for the "asexual feminine nature" observed by some writers). It might also be defined as the inability to completely give oneself sexually. Parenthetically, unless a woman is able to make a full emotional surrender, she will be sexually unfulfilled, a point of crucial importance and one which we will expand in subsequent chapters.

Why will a wife so often refuse to *give?* Because she has been taught that she should not do so, that giving is always a capitulation and hence a defeat. And, ironically, she has been taught that she will lose something of her womanhood by such giving. The irony, of course, is that by not fully giving she loses all opportunity to attain womanhood.

In our society, virtually every wife has been exposed to a Ph.D. education in this philosophy. Essentially, she is indoctrinated in anti-masculinism and anti-sexualism. And calling it *indoctrination* hardly seems an exaggeration! Consider, if you will, what a girl is subjected to as she struggles to mature and to discover who and what she is. Initially, she may hear cynical, if not bitter, comments on men and marriage from a dissatisfied mother. Often, this "teaching" is very subtle. It may be more an impression that is conveyed rather than anything explicit. Her mother may approach life with a resignation which emphasizes the "sacrificial" nature of the woman's role and thereby convey the feeling that there is nothing desirable in being born female. How many times, for example, does a girl listen to remarks about it being a "man's world." And how many times is she told that she cannot take part in certain activities because "that's for boys." More often than not, these are the words of her mother. Multiply them by thousands throughout her childhood, and the result becomes apparent: she will enter marriage feeling resentment and hostility, even if she is unable to verbalize it or admit it to herself. She will resent the submissive role of the wife and the dominant role of the husband. And resentment can only breed hostility. The hostility, however, is directed more toward herself than toward her husband; she doesn't like being a woman—ergo, she doesn't like herself. What she feels toward men is, thus, partly owing to her feelings of self-contempt (emotional defenses) and partly to the distorted image she has been given of men, women, and marriage.

The effect such mothers have in shaping their daughter's attitudes—and lives—is great. The influence would be less potent, however, if it were not for the strong support and reinforcement it receives from the many forces supplying munitions for a war between the sexes. But "war between the sexes" is perhaps not the best description of the conflict, for while there may be some surface animosity between men and women, the campaign is directed more toward a denial of sexual differences. It will have succeeded when it is no longer possible to distinguish men from women! Does the statement seem extreme? In one recent book attacking the traditional role of the Christian wife, the author contends that sexual relations are more satisfying if the spouses are able to ignore their sexual differences!

Those who are striving to desexualize (and hence, dehumanize) men and women generally talk a great deal about *equality* of the sexes. This has been the dominant *cause célèbre* of the feminists since the inception of the movement in eighteenth-century England. Great strides have been made and continue to be made toward eliminating the inequities which existed and which still exist. But while these efforts were initially directed against discrimination in employment, education, and suffrage, they have now generalized to include the relationship of husband and wife. Wives are repeatedly being told that they must declare their independence and assert their right to equality. (One of the favorite catch-phrases of the protagonists is "Women must first be accepted as persons." But can one be a *person* without being a man or woman?) It has become the theme and the rallying cry of the women's magazines (with sophomoric love stories and recipes sandwiched in between) and the perennial topic for panel discussions and neighborhood coffee klatches, all of which reinforces the role teaching of the embittered mothers of many contemporary wives.

What was called *feminism* in the 1920s is now "woman's quest for identity"; the anti-masculinism of the suffragettes has been muted; now, the neo-feminists speak of the "feminine mystique." Only the words have changed, however. The stereotyping of the sexes (always negative), the hostility toward marriage, the resentment at not having been born male, all are still present. And, if a wife is to gain the freedom to become a woman, she must be constantly on guard against an influence which has increased in its insidiousness as it has increased in subtlety.

Again, the word *freedom.* If the words *strength* and *responsibility* typify a man, the word *freedom* seems especially fitting to describe a woman. Finding her fulfillment in marriage, she is free to be a *woman,* free, that is to *love.* A short time ago, we listened to a group of college undergraduates in a round-table discussion of engagement and marriage. One particularly bright girl showed a remarkable understanding of womanhood when she said, "Women have a real advantage over men. You men have to be concerned with a number of specific responsibilities in your job, in the community, and in your family. As a wife, only one thing is demanded of a woman: she must be always *ready.*" What she meant by this, she went on to explain, is that a wife must be flexible in her moods and responses so that she is at all times "ready" to respond to her husband, to love him in the ways in which he needs to be loved *at that moment.* No book can tell the ways in which to love. At one time it may be by offering support, or perhaps just an accepting ear. At another time, it may be by letting her husband know of her trust. And still another time, she may best love by remaining silent. The goal for a communication system between husband and wife should always be the understanding of the emotional needs of the other.

This, of course, is an obligation which applies to both spouses. The wife, however, has an advantage. The meaning of her whole vocation is found in loving. And her vocation—to love—is also her nature. Truly, the wife is the "heart of the family." And, like the body, marriage needs but one "head" and one "heart"; both, functioning within their nature, are indispensable.

Dr. Marie N. Robinson has described the "essential feminine altruism" which characterizes a woman. As she points out, this need to give "the very best of herself" to her husband and children is rooted in the biology of woman; it is the hallmark of her nature. This is not a mere willingness to give of herself; it is an inherent *need* to give. Should she be deprived of an outlet for her altruistic need or refuse to express it, she will nurture the seeds of frustration which some feel is the chronic unnamed illness of the contemporary wife.

This altruism, this desire to give herself to her family, has a dramatic effect on a woman; we might say it transforms her into a woman. More than all else, it is the quality which makes the eternal woman enigmatic. Most husbands (and, unfortunately, many wives) find it impossible to understand how a woman can cope with the myriad demands, large and small, made each day by children and the never-ending task of maintaining a home. The wife who has attained womanhood is able to do something more than merely cope with these demands, however; she is able to find joy and humor in doing so. She finds humor in her family, in the world about her, and most of all, in herself. Her givingness underlies the pervasive tranquility which is the beauty, and the enigma, of a woman. She radiates it. And it motivates her to reach out to others in order to share the joy she has found. She does this with an enthusiasm which is infectious. Like the child discovering a small world of wildflowers, she seems almost breathless in her eagerness to share the excitement she finds in being a woman.

Not that she is immune to the pressures arising from the demands made upon her. She, too, can lose her composure; she can show anger, feel sadness, experience frustration.

But it isn't a lasting thing. She doesn't go on day after day destroying herself and her marriage with her bitterness. Neither is she torn apart with anxiety. The fact that so many wives suffer from countless fears may, in truth, be more indicative of a lack of womanhood than a reflection of reality factors. In loving, she places her complete trust in her husband and, through him, in God. Hence, her faith is an expression of her love. And it is in this love that her fear dissolves.

A love which is expressed in a total reliance upon another is an ideal not easily attained. And it can be tricky. All the reasons we give ourselves to justify not loving are so self-satisfying and so "sensible" that we often fail to recognize their self-deception. Furthermore, a refusal to love increases our own misery, and, in an effort to relieve our unhappiness, we fall into even more egocentric behavior. How often we say, "These are the reasons why I can't love him (or her)," when it would be more honest if we were to admit, "These are the opportunities I have been given to love—and won't!" The ever-present temptation is to evaluate—judge, if you will—whether the other one is loving us. But if, at any time, we concern ourselves with *being loved,* we can be sure of only one thing: *We are failing to love!*

We have said that sexuality is not merely some part of marriage, that the entire relationship is sexual; it is the relationship of a man and woman. In the life of a wife, seldom is the extent of her willingness to give more evident than in the manner in which she approaches the marital union. As she becomes more a woman, the meaning of the sexual embrace becomes clearer to her. Rather than viewing it as a male prerogative, she gratefully accepts her own sexual enjoyment. Here, too, she follows his lead. She neither makes sexual demands, seeking satisfaction when and how it suits her, nor sets limits on their sexual love.

Assuming there is no violation of morality involved (which, of course, would negate loving), she is ready and eager to love him in the ways in which he desires to be loved, and, in doing so, she quickly discovers that they are the ways in which she, too, wishes to make love.

In their sexual relations, as in all else, they are equals. They each give and receive without demands, without exploitation, and without resentment. Sexually, the marital *rights* are the rights to love and be loved in the most intimate and meaningful of human encounters. And this applies to both. But they love and are loved in different, yet complementary, ways. As a wife comes to a realization of her responsibilities and her nature, she discovers a very important truth: that she can become a *woman*, and that any woman can become fully a *woman*, only through a man. This is as true of a nun as it is of a married woman, a truth which is recognized when a nun accepts the wedding band and pledges her life to her spouse, Christ—a man. For the Christian wife, the wife who has grown into womanhood, there is no rivalry. What she freely gives to her husband, she gives to herself: the splendor promised in Eden. She becomes him, they become one, and she becomes fully a woman.

It may seem that we are saying that a wife must step off a cliff in order to become a woman, that she must throw herself into the arms of her husband and Providence. We are! Is this foolish? Of course! Unrealistic? Perhaps. But possible? Yes, since it is of the nature of a woman, and the essence of loving. And hence, it embodies the meaning of Christianity. And there is nothing so foolish or unrealistic as Christianity—unless the good news of Christ's redemptive love is true!

CHAPTER V

Sexual Anatomy of Man

IN LOWER ANIMALS, the sexual union is largely an instinctual act. At maturity, stimuli specific to the species trigger the behavior which initiates mating. These are unlearned patterns of behavior, occurring alike in all members of a species, patterns which are serviceably complete on the occasion of their first appearance. No course of instruction or tutoring in the facts of life is necessary. If man, however, at one time had these innate responses, they have long been buried in his evolutionary past. Human sexual roles must be learned. The physical state of sexual arousal occurs in all normal human beings, but the intended functioning of our sexual faculties is not something which is immediately apparent. A certain amount of instruction is necessary.

For a society which has so often been accused of being obsessed with sex, ignorance of the essential "facts" of sexuality might be thought to be a thing of the past. Unfortunately, however, we still see many couples who enter marriage with little or no knowledge of the reproductive functions of man and woman. Often such lack of information will be coupled with many unhealthy attitudes.

Only in humans can the sexual act become an act of love. Sexual relations in marriage can develop in variety and meaning and can express the deepest human emotions. In order for such loving to mature, however, there must exist both the desire to sexually love—to give oneself to meet the emotional needs of the other—and knowledge: knowledge of one's spouse, and knowledge of the basic physical make-up of man and woman.

Anatomy is the department of biology which deals with the form and structure of organisms and their parts, that is, the composition and structural relations of the parts. Physiology may be said to be the sister of anatomy. It is the branch of science which studies the functions of organisms, the purposes served by the various organs, the way in which the various parts work, and the laws which govern their functions. And, ultimately, it is the study of the activities of the body as a whole. Any study of physiology must always be related to anatomy since, in order to understand the functioning of the body and its parts, we must have something of a picture of the organism.

We said these scientific disciplines are branches of biology; and, as we subdivide science, they are. But they also might appropriately be taught in an introductory course in theology. As we study the intricate design and complex functioning of the human body, we are continually awed by its beauty and by the glory it gives to its Creator. A pathologist with a lifetime of experience expressed it well when he said: "It has never been difficult for me to believe in God; I have spent my life studying His work." A recognition of the beauty of the reproductive mechanism is part of the recognition of the beauty of sexuality.

Frequently, books on marriage will present the anatomy and physiology of sex as if solely the organs of reproduction were involved. This can be misleading. The human sexual apparatus encompasses far more than the genital organs and certain related parts. While the reproductive system is the only system which is not necessary to the survival of the organism, it is at least as complex as the other bodily systems. Furthermore, all other systems, digestion, respiration, circulation, etc., play important roles in reproduction. If we go a step further and expand the discussion to take in the physiology of *sexuality*, we find our topic encompasses nearly the entire body.

Needless to say, such an undertaking is not our intention. On the other hand, any discussion of the anatomy and physiology of sex must extend beyond the organs of reproduction. In fact, it seems appropriate to start not with discussion of the sexual organs, but with the nervous system.

The body's communication network, the nervous system, is usually categorically divided into the *central* and *peripheral* nervous systems. This division does not denote that they are separate in their functioning. It is merely for expository purposes. The central nervous system includes the brain and spinal cord. Branching out from the brain and spinal cord, somewhat similar to the root distribution of a tree, are the cranial and spinal nerves. Together with their combinations and the peripheral portions of the autonomic nervous system, they comprise the peripheral nervous system.

At the extreme branches of the peripheral nervous system, the sense receptors and the special sense organs form our link with the outside world. Stimulation of these receptors causes an impulse to travel a sensory nerve pathway and conduct sensation from the various body areas or the special sense organs to the spinal cord and brain. Essentially, this is an input system, sending information about our environment to the brain. The brain, like a computer (only far more sophisticated than even the most advanced mechanical "brain") synthesizes and abstracts the incoming information, draws upon a vast storehouse of memories, associations, and responses, and "perceives" the nature and quality of the incoming signal.

Signals, in return, are sent by the central nervous system to the muscles and control their contraction and relaxation and, hence, voluntary movement. All of our purposive actions, from repairing a watch to making love, are dependent upon this two-way communication system.

In addition to these voluntary movements, there are many physiological processes of which we are usually unaware. Secretion of certain glands, heartbeat, constriction of peripheral blood vessels, and control of the muscle of the gastrointestinal tract walls are some of the functions of a special nerve network, the *autonomic nervous system*. These various involuntary processes (the *visceral* activities) are controlled, directly or indirectly, through the two divisons of the autonomic nervous system, the *parasympathetic* system and the *sympathetic* system. These two "sub-systems" act to check and balance each other in many of their functions. While we still have much to learn about the autonomic nervous system, it is known that the physiological reactions associated with emotion (release of epinephrine into the bloodstream, rise in blood pressure, increased cardiac output, increased blood sugar, increased oxygen consumption, sweating, etc.) all implicate the sympathetic system, and that these reactions generally also occur in response to sexual activity.

Our thoughts, perceptions, associations, and learned responses play a major role in our sexual behavior. These all involve the so-called higher brain centers. We as yet know little of the complex physiology of these mental activities. We do know, however, that maximal sexual arousal—and satisfaction—is dependent upon a combination of such higher mental activity, sensory input from the various sensory modalities, and sensations arising from tactile stimulation of the genitals.

Of major importance in sexual functioning, as well as in the development of the physical and emotional characteristics which comprise what we describe as the *nature* of man or woman, are the secretions of several hormone-producing glands. These *endocrine,* or ductless, glands act in concert to determine body growth and development, distribution of fatty tissue, secondary sex characteristics, hair distribution and complexion, pitch of voice, and energy. They also directly or indirectly influence the development of our personality. In addition to the sex glands, or *gonads* (testicles in the male and ovaries in the female), the endocrine system includes the pituitary, thyroid, parathyroid, adrenal, thymus, pancreas, and pineal glands. Stimulated by the autonomic nervous system and by an intricate feedback mechanism involving the biochemistry of the whole body, these hormone-producing glands are vital to the individual's well being as well as his behavior.

Hormone secretion may affect sexual performance in several ways. First of all, hormones released into the bloodstream may stimulate centers in the central nervous system which lead to sexual arousal; secondly, they affect the growth and development of the reproductive organs and the development of secondary sex characteristics; and, finally, they greatly affect general health and level of energy and this, in turn, affects sexual activity.

In addition to the proper functioning of these "essential" systems, healthy sexual functioning depends upon healthy functioning of the entire body. Proper functioning of the alimentary, excretory, respiratory, and circulatory systems, as well as the nervous and muscular systems is essential to healthy sexual performance.

The external male reproductive organs consist of the *penis* and the *testes* (or *testicles*). The penis is a highly complex organ which serves a twofold function of transporting urine out of the body and conducting semen, during the marital union, into the vaginal passage of the female. The organ forms a protective covering for the urogenital passage through which both urine and semen are discharged from a slit opening (the *meatus*) at the end of the organ. If we could look at a cross-section of the penis, we would observe three major divisions or parts extending lengthwise through it. The bulk of the penis is occupied by the two *corpora cavernosa*. These long muscular columns are unique both in structure and function. Essentially, they operate sexually as a hydraulic system. They are traversed by many blood channels. Ordinarily, these cavities are collapsed. Under sexual arousal, however, they rapidly fill with blood, creating a pressure which causes the penis to enlarge and become erect and firm. The stiff, erect, condition of the organ assures the ejection of the male seed deep within the vaginal receptable of the woman. With erection, it may swell to nearly twice its usual (flaccid) length and diameter. Valves, like floodgates that can be shut, prevent the return flow of blood and maintain the erection. A third, smaller, muscle column, the *corpus spongiosum*, extends along the back of the penis and surrounds and protects the urethra.

The gross structure of the penis includes the head of the organ, the *glans;* a rim at the base of the glans, the *corona;* the main body, or *shaft,* which forms most of its length; and the base of the penis where it joins the body. The glans is abundantly supplied with nerve endings and hence is usually the most sensitive part of the penis to erotic stimulation.

A fold of skin, the *prepuce,* partially covers the glans. Also called the foreskin, it is frequently removed surgically either because it is too long or too tight or, more commonly, as a hygienic measure (there are glands on or near the inside ridge of the glans which secrete a substance, *smegma,* that tends to accumulate and cause irritation). This minor operation, *circumcision,* also has religious significance. The distinguishing mark of the Chosen People, it was demanded by God in His covenant with Abraham: *You shall circumcise the flesh of your foreskin; it shall be a token of the covenant between you and Me* (Gen. 18:11). Christ's submission to the Covenant of Abraham, the first shedding of His blood, is celebrated as a major feast day of the Church on the first of January.

The testes (testicles) are a pair of oval bodies about an inch and a half in length. In the normal adult male, they lie in the scrotum, a thin-walled sac with two compartments hanging underneath the penis. During the embryonic stage of life, the testes develop within the abdominal cavity. The male sex cells, however, cannot grow in the warmer body heat of the abdomen. Shortly before birth, or occasionally later, the testes descend into the cooler environment of the scrotum. Should they fail to descend, the man will be sterile.

The testes serve a dual function: they are the sole site of development of sperm, or spermatozoa, the male sex cell by which the female may be impregnated; and they secrete the male sex hormone, *testosterone.* The hormone production is a function of special cells, Leydig cells, found in the supporting tissue. The testes, however, are not the only producers of male sex hormones. The adrenals also, in lesser amounts, secrete hormones associated with male characteristics.

The sperm develop in long convoluted tubules. When mature, they move into collecting tubules and on to the *epididymis,* a group of ducts which lie along one side of each testicle and act as a storehouse for the sperm. The epididymis also affects the functioning of the sperm. The fully grown sperm which emerge from the testicles are microscopic in size, smaller than most cells in the body, and unique in appearance. They have an ovoid, solid "head," containing the chromosomes, the genetic legacy from the father, and a long whiplike tail for propulsion, giving them an appearance not unlike polliwogs. In the testes, however, the sperm are unable to propel themselves. The ability to "swim" is acquired in the epididymis. This ability is very important; it enables the sperm to penetrate the uterus and Fallopian tubes of the woman to fertilize the female egg.

The *vas deferens* is continuous with the epididymis. Through it the semen is conveyed up through the inguinal canal to the urethra. This fluid contains much more than sperm. Along its journey from the testes, it is added to by the secretions from several glands.

Two glands which make a major contribution to the final composite seminal fluid are the *seminal vesicles* and the *prostate*. The two seminal vesicles are convoluted sacs which lie beneath the urinary bladder and behind the neck of the bladder. They secrete a sticky fluid which forms the major part of the semen. This fluid is alkaline and serves to protect the sperm, the sperm being unable to survive in an acid environment. The prostate is the largest accessory male sex structure. This heart-shaped organ encircles the urethra just below the bladder. It is believed that it aids the motility of the sperm by neutralizing its acid suspension and hence increases the likelihood of impregnation.

Ejaculation, the emission of semen from the penis, is essentially a reflex reaction. Impulses arising in the genitals, particularly the glans, are transmitted to the spinal cord and brain, built up to a peak, and set off returning nerve impulses which stimulate the emission of semen and the sensations known as the orgasm.

Hence, the final culmination of the male sex act results from a series of psychological and physiological events, actions, and reactions. Signals arising in the brain are transmitted to the genitals. Sensations in the genital organs are, in turn, sent to the spinal cord and on to the brain. Lubricating glands discharge into the urethra. Secretions from the prostate enter the urethra and alkalinize the semen. The seminal vesicles secrete their substance to add to the total discharge. From the vas deferens, the sperm enter the urethra. Finally, by a convulsive contraction of the muscles in the penis, this combined seminal fluid is forcefully discharged. This fluid, the *ejaculate*, has a total quantity of usually three to four mililiter, or about a teaspoon. It contains an amazing number of sperm, normally 120 to 150 million permililiter—or a total of about 500 million sperm!

Since only a single sperm impregnates the female egg, why are a half-billion ejaculated? We don't know. But what a beautiful mystery to ponder: that single tiny cell carries the curly hair, the brown eyes, and the broad shoulders of the father as God permits man and woman to share in His love and co-operate in His plan for the continuation of the species.

CHAPTER VI

Sexual Anatomy of Woman

IN GOD'S PLAN for the continuation of the species, the male has only a single function: he produces the male seed, the spermatozoa, and implants it within the body of the female. The body of a woman, on the other hand, is designed to: (a) produce the female egg, (b) provide the environment in which the impregnated egg, an embryonic human being, can develop, and (c) nurture, with food produced by her body, the new-born infant. Previously we said that woman's sexuality touches all of her *being*. On the physical level, it touches nearly all of her body. Its development profoundly affects her personality. Its cyclical variations affect her moods. Embracing her physical sexuality, and living in harmony with it, she matures into womanhood.

In the preceding chapter we briefly outlined the roles of the nervous and endocrine systems in the development and functioning of the male reproductive organs. In some respects, the interaction of these systems is more complex in the female. For one thing, the normal adult male functions reproductively in a somewhat constant manner. The testes are continually producing sperm which are then either discharged from the body or absorbed. The female, on the other hand, undergoes a dramatic physiological cycle approximately every lunar month. From the onset of puberty until middle age, when she is not carrying a child her body each month prepares for conception.

The functioning of this cycle can probably be best explained if we start with a brief description of the female sexual anatomy.

The female reproduction system can be grossly divided into internal and external organs of generation. The internal organs are the *ovaries*, the *Fallopian tubes*, the *uterus*, and the *vagina*. The external genitals are collectively called the *vulva* and include all of the reproductive tract visible from without.

The ovaries are a pair of structures located on either side of the uterus, or womb, near its upper end. They are almond shaped organs about an inch to an inch and a half in length, an inch in width, and about a quarter of an inch in thickness. From each ovary, a passageway leads to the uterus. These are the Fallopian tubes. At the other end, each Fallopian tube opens into the uterus.

The uterus is a thick-walled, hollow, muscular organ suspended in the pelvic cavity. It is pear-shaped, with its narrow end pointing downward. It lies between the bladder in front and the rectum behind. When not pregnant, the normal uterus is about three inches long, two inches wide, and an inch thick. During pregnancy, when the child is developing within its walls, the uterus rapidly increases in size and weight, reaching a length of eight inches and a weight of as much as two pounds. Following delivery, the uterus gradually resumes its original size and shape. It is the powerful contractions of the uterine walls that constitute what are called labor pains; and it is these muscular contractions which expel the baby at the time of delivery into the birth canal.

The vagina, or birth canal, is a sheath. In fact, the word *vagina* means sheath. It is a passageway leading from the vulva to the *cervix*, the neck of the uterus. Normally it is about three and a half inches in length. The walls of the vagina, however, are elastic in a longitudinal, as well as transverse, direction and hence even a large penis can usually penetrate to its length during intercourse. The vagina serves three principal functions: (a) It receives the male penis during sexual relations; (b) It serves as the outlet for the menstrual flow; (c) It serves as the birth canal through which the baby passes at birth.

The vagina extends downward and forward. Its walls are lined with a soft tissue resembling mucous membrane. It differs from mucous membrane, however, in that it does not contain secreting glands. Near the opening of the vagina are the *glands of Bartholin*, which, together with glands in the cervix, provide a fluid which lubricates the vagina during sexual stimulation. At its lower end, it is encircled with muscles which may be active during sexual intercourse.

The external opening of the vagina is relatively more contracted. In the virgin, the vaginal opening may be partly closed by a thin membrane, the *hymen*, which extends from the posterior wall in a crescent shape. Since the hymen is usually torn or stretched during initial intercourse, its presence intact has long been considered a proof of virginity. It is now generally recognized, however, that the presence or absence of this membrane can provide no such definite evidence of virginity. Often, the hymen is stretched or torn in childhood by accident. It may also be ruptured during medical examination or even surgically removed where, in rare cases, it completely closes the passageway and hence prevents the discharge of menstrual flow. On the other hand, sexual intercourse in some cases results in the hymen being stretched but not torn; thus it may retain the appearance of virginity. In the physical examination which should be included in the marriage preparations of both husband and wife, the physician can determine if the hymen, because of thickness or rigidity, is apt to cause difficulty in initial intercourse and, if so, can remedy the difficulty.

The external genital organs in the woman extend from the round fatty eminence above the pubic bone, the *mons veneris*, to the area between the rectum and the vagina. Enclosing the vulva are two longitudinal folds of skin, the *labia majora* (large lips). They are skin-colored and are covered with hair on their outer surface. These lips usually touch in the virgin. After repeated sexual experience, however, and especially following childbirth, they may not form as complete a closure. They form a protective enclosure for the more sensitive tissues and organs they cover.

Between the labia majora are a second, smaller, set of lips, the *labia minora* (small lips). They meet at the front of the vulva and are thinner than the labia majora, which makes it possible for them to be protected within the folds of the larger lips. These smaller lips are more pronounced in front, lessening in size toward the rear until they finally disappear in the posterior portions of the labia majora. In appearance and texture, they resemble the inner surface of the labia majora. Both are soft and smooth, pink in color, and slightly moist. The inner surfaces of the smaller lips are normally in contact. When the woman is sexually aroused, they tend to become distended with blood and increasingly sensitive. During the act of sexual intercourse, they act to guide the penis into the vagina. Toward the forward end of the vulva, the smaller lips join to form a small ridge just beneath a small, but sexually very important, structure, the *clitoris*.

The clitoris is an organ not unlike the penis in shape, but much smaller. It varies in length, but is usually three quarters of an inch to one and a half inches long. Most of the organ is concealed beneath the surface; only the upper end, the *glans,* is exposed.

In addition to appearance, the clitoris resembles the penis in sexual sensitivity. The glans of the clitoris, like the glans of the penis, has a heavy concentration of nerve endings, far more than the vagina. This finding has, in part, led to a major controversy. Many sexologists have viewed the clitoris as if it were nearly an exact homologue of the penis. They contend that the glans is the seat of sexual pleasure—and orgasm—in woman. While conceding that other parts of the genitalia are capable of erotic feeling, they claim that it is solely in the head of the clitoris that the sexual climax is experienced. Others have concluded that the so-called "clitoral orgasm" reflects an earlier phylogenetic period and an elementary stage in sexual maturation. They are convinced that the sexually mature woman is not only capable of experiencing orgasm through vaginal stimulation alone (that is, stimulation by the penis during coitus), but that "vaginal orgasm" is a deeper and more meaningful experience. If the question involved nothing more than a rather trivial point of physiology, we could easily dismiss it. Its implications, however, extend much further. In fact, the clitoral versus vaginal orgasm controversy touches on some of the pivotal assumptions underlying the marital union. Because the question seems less physical than psychological or philosophical, we will postpone further examination of it (see Chapter IX).

The clitoris resembles the penis in yet another way: it is composed mostly of erectile tissue, capable of suffusion and distention by the inflow of blood, and thus, like the penis, reaches a state of erection during sexual arousal.

In at least one major respect, these male and female organs differ. Unlike the penis, the clitoris does not enclose the urethra for the passage of urine. The female urethra emerges below the clitoris and is a much shorter passage from the bladder.

The *mammary glands,* or breasts, are properly included among the organs of the female reproductive system. Since they are not directly concerned in reproduction, however, they are often referred to as accessory organs of the system. Before puberty, they are undeveloped and are essentially the same in appearance for both sexes. At puberty, a girl's breasts begins to increase in size and undergo a series of rapid changes. They grow larger during pregnancy and are usually largest during the period of nursing.

Near the center of each breast, or slightly below the center, is the outlet for the mother's milk, the nipple. This small conical eminence is surrounded by a slightly raised area of somewhat wrinkled skin, the *areola.* In younger women, this area is usually pinkish or crimson in color; it is usually darker in brunettes than in blondes. With pregnancy, this pigmented area enlarges and takes on a brownish color, a condition which remains after she gives birth. The female breasts, and particularly the nipples, are highly responsive to sexual stimulation. When sexually aroused, the nipples swell and become erect.

With this brief sketch of the sexual anatomy of woman, we can now discuss her sexual physiology.

The sexual cycle in woman is initiated and regulated by a small gland, about the size of a marble, situated behind the eyes and beneath the base of the brain, the *pituitary* gland. Actually, this gland is divided into two functionally distinct parts, the anterior and posterior pituitary. Only the anterior pituitary has a direct effect on sexual functioning. This organ secretes at least six different known hormones; some believe it may produce even more. Three of these are *gonadotrophic* hormones, so-called because they regulate the functions of the sexual glands. They are the *follicle stimulating hormone*, the *luteinizing hormone*, and the *luteotrophic hormone*.

When a girl reaches puberty, the pituitary gland begins secreting the gonadotrophic hormones. Not all at the same time, however. At first, only the follicle stimulating hormone is secreted. It sets in motion the sexual cycle of the adolescent girl.

Most of the approximately 100,000 or so ova (some have estimated as many as 400,000) that are formed during a woman's lifetime are present in the substance of the ovaries at birth, although they remain dormant until puberty. Each ovum is surrounded by a layer of special cells. Together, they make up what is called a *primary follicle*. The follicle-stimulating hormone causes a few of these to begin growing each month. The special outer layer of cells of the primary follicles in turn start to produce and secrete one of the two major female sex hormones, *estrogens*.

Together with the other ovarian hormone, *progesterone*, the estrogens are responsible for the sexual development of the female and also for her monthly sexual cycle.

The estrogens cause proliferation (increase in number) of many cells in the body, resulting in the development of the female sexual characteristics. Development of the breasts, growth of pubic hair, enlargement of the vagina and uterus, broadening of the hips, and the deposits of fatty tissue which give a woman her characteristic shape, are all brought about by the estrogens. In short, the estrogens physically transform a girl into a woman.

When the follicles which have started growing reach about one half their maximum size, the pituitary stops secreting follicle-stimulating hormone and begins to secrete luteinizing hormone. This hormone causes one of the follicles to increase greatly in size until finally it ruptures, expelling the ovum into the Fallopian tube. This monthly process is known as ovulation, and it is important that we understand something of how it takes place, since only then can we grasp how conception occurs. Ordinarily, only a single ovum is expelled each month, and it is during this period only that a woman can become pregnant. This is in sharp contrast with the billions of sperm that may be produced and expelled by a man during a comparable period.

Following its rupture, the follicle continues to grow in size. It develops a fatty, yellow appearance. For this reason, the entire mass of cells is called a *corpus luteum*—a "yellow body." It continues to develop and produces substances which act to build up the endometrium, the lining of the uterus, to prepare the womb to receive the fertilized ovum, should conception occur.

The third gonadotrophic hormone, *luteotrophic hormone*, is secreted by the pituitary about the time the follicle ruptures. It continues to be secreted for about two weeks. In addition to aiding the development of the follicular cells into lutein cells, it stimulates these cells to produce female sex hormones.

If pregnancy does not occur, the corpus luteum ceases to function and the endometrial tissues lining the uterine walls die and are sloughed off into the uterine cavity. This is the process known as *menstruation*.

The sperm fertilizes the ovum in the Fallopian tube and the fertilized egg then moves down and attaches itself to the wall of the uterus. It can be fertilized only during the period eight to twenty-four hours following ovulation. Similarly, the sperm can only live in the female for about twenty-four hours. Hence, for conception to take place, it is necessary that sexual relations occur either shortly before ovulation or within a few hours following it.

Ovulation ordinarily occurs on the fourteenth day of a twenty-eight-day cycle. The so-called Rhythm Method, employed either to increase the probability of conception or to prevent it, is based upon this fact. If conception is not felt to be advisable, abstinence from sexual relations during the four- or five-day period preceding ovulation is usually successful in preventing fertilization. Many women, however, have an irregular cycle, making it difficult to accurately estimate the time of ovulation. In such cases, the woman's physician may instruct her in a method of determining the time of ovulation based upon a deviation in body temperature which normally accompanies ovulation.

In women, there is nothing which corresponds to the ejaculation. The ovum is ejected on a schedule; the sperm is usually ejected reflexively as a result of sexual stimulation. Both, however, experience orgasm, and in both man and woman the event is marked by dramatic physical as well as psychological reactions.

CHAPTER VII

Love-making

LOVE IS the act of giving one's self. Love-making is the *art* of giving one's self—sexually. As with all art, it is the use of skill and imagination to produce something of beauty. Its beauty is the miracle of unity—"that two shall become one."

Beauty emerges within context, the setting natural to it. The human eye, for all its beauty, plucked from the setting of the face, becomes a thing of horror. The art of love-making, within the setting of which it is so much a part and for which it is intended, has a beauty surpassing all the treasures in the Louvre. Its setting is Christian marriage.

In all art, the artist must learn his medium. And he must acquire skill if he is to produce something truly of beauty. In love-making, the artistic medium is the body and all its faculties; her medium is his body, and his medium is her body. Their skill grows from an understanding of each other's "sexual anatomy," and from a ceaseless striving to perfect their love-making art.

With the onset of puberty, the child "comes of age." Almost overnight, people and things take on a new appearance. Dramatic physical changes are accompanied by painful awkwardness and a growing awareness of self, and of self-in-relation-to-others. For the first time, members of the opposite sex are seen *as opposite*—very strange creatures, indeed. And yet, somehow attractive. Gradually, powerful new urges filter through to consciousness, and the child steps across the threshold into the adult world. The experience is never free of anxiety, and seldom without conflict.

The tensions the child experiences during this period result from both physical and social changes. The developing sexual characteristics, the clashes with parents as the child seeks independence, the painful unsureness of first dates, all contribute to these tensions. But it is the growing experience of sexual arousal which most frequently lies at the core of adolescent anxiety.

Sexual arousal doesn't commence, however, with puberty; it merely becomes more pronounced and demanding. Even before the infant takes its first step, it experiences feelings which may properly be called sexual responses. We frequently, for example, observe an erection in baby boys of only a few months. There is a difference, however. At that age, the arousal reaction is reflexive in nature. It results from little more than tactile stimulation of the genitals.

By the time the child reaches puberty, many experiences and perceptions have become assoicated with the sexual arousal state. These learned associations form the major stimuli for the adult erotic response. Nearly any perception—a sight, a touch, a sound—can become a cue to elicit a sexual response. These early associations also determine many of our sexual preferences, the color of eyes we find appealing, the wavy hair, the tapered fingers. It is largely these associations which account for a boy being attracted to a girl who has the blue eyes of his mother, or a girl becoming infatuated with a man who smokes the same brand of pipe tobacco as her father.

In order to understand something of the psychological mechanisms of sexual arousal and its role in the love-making of marriage, we must understand the basic nature of our sex drive, and how our various senses serve to initiate and direct it.

The various physical drives, such as hunger and thirst, are states of tension. And like any tension states, they serve to activate the organism. It is this increasing tension which motivates us to seek satisfaction of the drive. Thus, we speak of the satisfaction of a drive as "tension reducing." The tension state associated with hunger is reduced by eating; the tension of thirst, by drinking, etc. But it is the *reduction* of the tension, and not the tension itself, which is satisfying. The tension itself gives no pleasure.

In the human sexual drive, however, we find something very different. Not only is the tension reduction of orgasm satisfying, the drive state of sexual arousal itself is pleasurable. Furthermore, it is usually pleasurable even when it is not ultimately terminated in orgasm.

It is important that this be understood since it touches upon the whole of human sexual activity and the purpose and meaning of sexuality in marriage. What is experienced in the mutual arousal of husband and wife is expressive of the deepest marital love. Through their actions and words, each strives to increase the sexual arousal—and pleasure—of the other. And it is this art of love-making which is truly the making of love.

The love-making which precedes coitus is frequently called *foreplay*. This is an unfortunate term, however, since it implies something other than mutual loving. It is a mistake to view pre-coital love-making as merely sexual arousing actions intended to bring the couple to a state of physical readiness for intercourse. And yet more than a few marriage manuals treat the subject solely in terms of instruction for husbands in techniques to be employed in bringing a wife to the point of physical readiness. They treat it as merely a means to an end, nothing more. Furthermore, they imply that it is only the husband who must arouse his partner, that he must engage in foreplay to "prepare" her for coitus. Often it is stated that men, being fully aroused in only a minute or two, have no need for preliminary love-making. Physically, if we are thinking solely in terms of achieving erection, this is true. But love-making is a mutual giving of self; and hence neither can assume a strictly passive role. And so, in loving her husband, the wife "makes love" by sexually stimulating him just as he gives the pleasure of sexual arousal to her.

It would also be a mistake to think of this love-making solely in terms of giving, even mutual giving. All love-making actions, regardless of how giving they may be, give pleasure and increasing arousal to the one giving—or at least this is the way it should be. This point may seem obvious, but it is often overlooked by those writing on marital sexuality. And it is too important a fact to be overlooked. The sexual arousal experienced by the one "giving" stems not only from observing the sexual response of the other one, but also from the physical stimulation experienced in the "giving." A husband, for example, may give intense pleasure to his wife by stimulating her breasts; at the same time, he will find her obvious pleasure very arousing. But more than this, he will experience strong sensations from stimulating her. Unless we keep this rather apparent fact in mind, we may tend to think of these love-making actions as solely *giving*, and overlook the pleasure that should be derived.

Love-making can never properly be divided into a sequence of periods or stages. Nor can we speak of a "beginning" or "end" of the love-making. To do so would lead us again into the error of splitting sexuality off from the rest of the marriage. Viewed in the context of the total relationship of husband and wife, we might realistically say that the husband initiates the love-making when he telephones from work during the day just to say, "I love you." Or that the wife makes the overtures when she devotes that extra five minutes to touching up her make-up before he arrives home. When we speak of foreplay, or of differing stages in marital relations, we should, therefore, keep in mind that the total sexual encounter is, properly, love-making, no part of which is merely preliminary to the making of love.

For expository purposes, however, we will discuss sexual arousal and love-making exclusive of the act of coitus, postponing discussion of the latter until the following chapter.

Each of our senses contributes to our total sexual arousal, or is at least capable of doing so. And the pleasure we experience is a composite of sensations from each of the sensory modalities. Sight, touch, smell, hearing, and taste work, to a great extent, in concert. At various moments during love-making, one of the senses may be predominant, but if we were deprived of any one of them— or if we were to inhibit any, whether because of faulty attitudes or because of uncertainty as to what is, or is not, a normal part of love-making—our enjoyment would be lessened and marital love would be impaired. In discussing each of the senses in turn, we do not, therefore, mean to imply that they can be viewed as functionally discrete.

Sight: Probably almost anything we are capable of seeing could become a stimulus for sexual arousal; all that would be necessary is a learned association between the object and the arousal state. Thus, a room, a flower, a picture, or a piece of clothing could become a sexual stimulus. Not all sights associated with sexual arousal, however, have the same strength as stimuli. Some may be only mildly arousing, while others may be very stimulating. And with some, there seem to be only what might be termed "indirect" associations with sexuality. These indirect, or *secondary*, visual stimuli are important, however. They form the romantic backdrop, what might be called the setting for love.

Most wives do not need to be told of the importance of romance. Romance, and the fantasies of romance, fills a great need in the life of a woman. Unfortunately, there are countless husbands who ignore this need, who approach sexual relations with little or no thought of romantic love. This, in fact, is so common an offense that many women assume that men are by nature unromantic.

As prevalent as this notion may be, it is nevertheless wholly unfounded. Men are innately no less romantic than women. But in our culture, men are frequently reluctant to admit romantic interests or express romantic love. They are taught to look with disdain at the stereotype of the continental lover. Kissing the lady's hand, sending the solitary rose, writing the love poem, are scorned as effeminate. And yet the romantic male lover is no less a *man* than the boorish husband who disregards his wife's desires. The unromantic husband does not evidence masculinity, only a lack of loving. Many husbands would do well to read the love stories published in popular women's magazines. As sophomoric as this fiction may be, it provides many women with at least the vicarious thrill of romantic love. And for a sizable number of them, this is the only romance that touches their lives.

Devoid of romance, however, sexual love becomes monotonous, unpleasant, and even exploitive. In other words, it ceases to be *love*. The wife feels "used" by her husband, resentful of his egocentric approach to sexual relations. One bitter wife spoke of the unromantic, matter-of-fact, manner in which her husband approached marital relations. As she talked with us, her frustration erupted in tears and hostility: "Sex? What is it to him? He doesn't love me; I'm just his sleeping pill!"

While women, at least by training, may have a stronger desire for secondary, or romantic, stimuli, it is the role of the man to set the romantic scene for the love-making. And this calls for awareness, imagination, and aesthetic sensibility. But, most of all, there must be a desire to love. He must structure an atmosphere of romance, one in which all the senses may be stimulated, acting in unison to enhance the total response of sexual love.

Does this mean that it is the husband only who is to be the lover, that the wife has no responsibilities for romance? Not at all. The home, as a setting for romance, is largely her responsibility. It need not have the appearance of a movie set or the bridal suite of a luxury hotel, but it can be romantic. The uncluttered room, the vase of flowers, the fresh bed linen, and the dab of perfume applied with love, can form a romantic backdrop for loving as exciting as the most exotic hideaway. In this regard, however, many wives fall short. They may complain of a lack of romance, but what husband can sustain feelings of romance with a wife who consistently retires with her hair in pin curls and wearing a flannel nightgown? And how long will the romance of the honeymoon last if she greets him each evening in housecoat and slippers or if she welcomes him home with a monotonous litany of minor gripes, trials, and tribulations—and the never-ending complaint of tiredness? The husband, however, is the wooer; his wife, the object of his wooing. Hence it is the husband, primarily, who assumes the lead, taking his cues from her spoken and unspoken desires, in the never-ending adventure of romantic love.

Any visually aesthetic scene may be described as a romantic setting. Our individual preferences, memories, and associations all play a part in determining what might be called the "romantic value" of a particular place. And, obviously, being in the company of the one we love may transform even the most familiar surrounding into one of romance. The husband who is intent on loving will seek to discover the settings most conducive to romance, the dinner by candlelight, the very private picnic for two, the stroll, hand in hand, on a moonlit beach. Like the violets he brings her when there is no "special occasion," these may correctly be called *secondary sexual stimuli*. By "secondary" is meant only that there is no necessary causal relationship between these stimuli and sexual arousal; we don't mean to imply that they are secondary in importance. We have asked many husbands, "When did you last take your wife on a date? Not out with friends or to some pre-arranged gathering, but just the two of you, for an evening that you planned for her?" Too often the answer is pathetic. Many husbands seem to associate dating only with courtship, or, at best, their dating efforts extended only through the honeymoon. But now married, they only occasionally "take the wife out," and usually these excursions have all the romance of a weekly shopping trip to the grocery. Out of ignorance or embarrassment, these husbands often dismiss suggestions of romance and see little relationship between romantic love and sexuality. In its influence on sexual responsiveness, however, most wives would give romance—and the love it conveys—a position of paramount importance. And for the loving husband, it will be no less so.

If husbands are often neglectful of these secondary stimuli, wives are as frequently unaware of the importance of *primary* visual stimulation in sexual arousal. Primary stimuli are those which are directly or causally associated with erotic response. While any object might, through association, become a primary stimulus, it is the sight of the nude or semi-nude body which usually is most arousing.

As human beings, we find pleasure in looking at attractive people—of both sexes. If love "makes the world go 'round," sex—in the image of the female form—causes the advertising agencies to rotate. Everything from elevator shoes to electron microscopes are promoted by provocative young females, a fact which has prompted more than a few social critics to accuse our society of sexual obsession.

The charge, however, does not seem justified, at least not on this evidence. To enjoy looking at an attractive girl is certainly not unnatural. We may question the morality of some of this advertising; and certainly a lot of it is in poor taste. In any case, it may be incongruous to employ a pretty girl to demonstrate a bulldozer, but the soundness of the psychology of such advertising can hardly be challenged.

We said that both sexes find enjoyment in looking at attractive members of the opposite sex. And yet the "sex appeal" in advertising is nearly all directed toward men; it is the female models who are dressed (or undressed) and posed most provocatively. Does this mean that women are not sexually stimulated by looking at the male form, or perhaps, even, that they are repelled by it? Of course not! Yet nevertheless, there are differences between the sexes in this regard, and these differences should be recognized and understood.

Observing these differences, some writers have gone to the extreme of stating that very few women are sexually aroused by the sight of the male body (but that men, on the other hand, find the undraped female very stimulating). While the statement is inaccurate, it's not difficult to understand how such a conclusion might be reached. Men's magazines, featuring fold-out color photographs of nude girls, enjoy large circulations; strip-tease dancers rate star billing; and a topless swim suit was pictorially featured in leading publications (prompting a few arrests and a number of letters to editors). But there is no similar public display of the male body. Even the male physique magazines have very few women readers. Nevertheless, there may be several explanations, other than a lack of feminine interest in the male body, to account for this. We might find most of the reasons by again examining the social influence. Our culture determines, or at least influences, what is (and is not) a sexual stimulus. In our society, boys are "taught" to be voyeuristic and girls are "taught" to be exhibitionistic. That is, it is socially expected that males will be stimulated by *looking* at the female body, and that females will enjoy, at least within limits, *displaying* their bodies to be looked at. But how much, if any, of this is innate and how much is a learned behavior we can probably never determine.

It is most surely incorrect, however, to conclude that a wife will not become sexually aroused by viewing her husband's nude body. Of course she will—assuming she loves her husband and has developed positive attitudes toward sexuality.

But some problems, we must admit, arise frequently enough to warrant some additional comment and at least a few hesitant generalizations about the sexes in this regard.

For one thing, we hear wives complain that their husbands look at "those pictures" in the men's magazines. These women often draw all kinds of inferences from this male interest in the female form. We have listened to them accuse their spouses of everything from perversity to adultery solely on this evidence. Yet seldom do these wives look at themselves to see what they are, or are not, doing. One happily married wife put her finger on at least a part of the problem: "These women want to know why their husbands enjoy watching strip-tease dancers and looking at pin-ups? It's because, as wives, they're misers."

There is a truth in her statement which applies to many wives. Self-righteously, they condemn the strip-tease dancers and the men who watch them, but just as self-righteously they refuse to disrobe or provocatively display their bodies before their husbands. The result is a sad irony: the pin-up models and the dancers, motivated by money, give something which these wives, who should be motivated by love, refuse to give!

This is not offered as a rationale, nor as a justification, for strip-tease dancing or girlie magazines. Nor are we making any attempt to explain their popularity on the basis of a lack of giving on the part of some wives. We feel sure the reasons extend much further than that, and there can probably be no single explanation for the growing phenomena of public nudity and commercial exploitation of sexuality. But many a wife would do well to recognize the importance of such primary sexual stimuli to her husband, and the ways in which she can enhance his sexual arousal—and hence love him—by casting off any inhibitions and false modesty (too often rationalized as a virtue) which prevent her from exhibiting her body to her husband.

We said false modesty, and the emphasis should be on the word *false*. Nudity between husband and wife has nothing—repeat, nothing—to do with the virtue of modesty. In the intimacy of marriage, undress for each other should be as natural and unself-conscious as a shared laugh or a mutual prayer.

Much can usually be done by the husband to help his wife overcome whatever embarrassment and reticence marital nudity may cause, especially in aiding her (and himself) during the early months of marriage when so much must usually be unlearned. He can give her the encouragement, the admiration, the security, and, in a word, the *love* which will make it possible for her to naturally and willingly reveal herself—emotionally as well as physically—to him. Without his encouragement, she can be expected to hold back. One husband, after twelve years of marriage, complained that his wife was seldom willing to disrobe in his presence. His wife freely admitted it and then went on to explain, "I've never been able to convince myself that he finds me attractive. Never once has he admired my shape, or said anything to indicate that he likes looking at me. Last Christmas, I asked him if, just once, he might give me some intimate, personal gift, rather than something for the house. And do you know what I received? A long flannel nightgown!"

We might say that he could learn a few things about how best to flatter a wife. A husband's gift of diaphanous lingerie will seldom fail to communicate a very important message. She may not have the measurements of a pin-up girl, but no matter. His gift tells her that he finds her sexually appealing, and, in a lovingly subtle manner, it gives her the cue that permits her to express, through the revealment of her body, her love for him.

False modesty interferes with the freedom of sexual love in still another way. Occasionally we find couples who have sexual relations only in the most secretive manner: at night, in bed, with the lights out. It's almost as if they feel that love-making is too shameful an act for the light of day, and too regulated by convention to be engaged in anywhere but in bed. This might not be the reason they would give, but what other reason might we infer? The question isn't whether making love in the afternoon is better than at night, or whether it's more enjoyable before an open fireplace than in bed, but whether or not they are able to fully enjoy the beauty of their bodies and freedom in their sexual love. Again, the word *freedom*. Unless they possess the emotional freedom to make love in the sunshine on a deserted beach, the love-making in the darkness of their bedroom will most likely be lacking.

Hearing: Just as candlelight can be a secondary visual stimulus, certain sounds can also become secondary stimuli for sexual arousal. Music, for example. The power of music as an erotic stimulant is so well recognized that little needs to be said. Some of the rigid anti-sexualists have even given it an importance as an aphrodisiac it doesn't merit. They raise alarms each time a new musical fad, such as rock-and-roll, captures the young. They warn youth of the captivating force of "hypnotic drums" and "savage rhythms." In other words, they view music as a primary, rather than secondary, stimulus.

Hopefully, few of us take these warnings seriously. Music may have charms to soothe the savage, but not to drive him to a sexual frenzy. Nevertheless, music can play an important part in influencing our emotional reactions. "Mood" music can affect, as well as reflect, our moods. Students of liturgical music have long recognized this. The music of the liturgy stirs the emotions of the faithful as well as giving glory to God. The music of the love song stirs the emotions of the lovers as well as giving love to each other.

We frequently speak of "background music." In love-making, this background may be formed by the beauty of the music and the mood suggested by the melody, by chordal progressions, by rhythmic patterns, or by the memories associated with the music—especially those shared by the couple. It may also be formed by the images the words of the song evoke.

Here again, most couples have memories of the romantic music of their courting days, those melodies that became theirs alone. These are the threads that make up the tapestry of romance. Why let it collect dust once they marry? Dancing to a recording in the living room, just the

two of you, should, if anything, be more romantic than it
was when you heard the song together for the first time.
Romance, though, can die unless the couple work to keep
it alive. Too many allow it to atrophy. They neglect the
sights and sounds of romance and permit their marriage to
become dull and routine; for them, the melody of the love
song becomes only a vague memory of a courtship that
should never have ended.

We might say that the history of the famous loves has
been written in verse and melody, beginning with the Song
of Songs. The poetry of love is both an avowal of love as
well as a source of arousal when made a part of the
romantic love of husband and wife. And it should be. Actually, the two should be inseparable since all acts and
words intended to be sexually arousing should also communicate love.

While erotic poetry such as Walter Benton's *This Is My
Beloved* has a proper place in a couple's repertoire of
love-making, it should not be necessary to rely upon the
words of a poet in order to verbally communicate sexual
love. The words of her husband expressing his love and his
desire for her should be far more stimulating to a wife than
the most exquisite love sonnet.

A free expression of sexual desires is not merely stimulating, it is imperative to the growth of sexual love. The
attainment of mutual satisfaction rests on such communication. And yet here many couples are sadly deficient.
Lack of good verbal communication plagues many marriages, and in no area of marriage is this more evident
than in discussion of sexuality.

A reluctance to talk about sexual feelings may be due to
embarrassment, or it may stem from the mistaken notion
that such talk, even between husband and wife, is somehow unseemly. It may also partly result from a limited
vocabulary of correct anatomical terms. Many husbands

know only vernacular words for the genitals and for sexual relations. And yet they feel that to use such words would be offensive. Like so many of our misconceptions, this one has become institutionalized. The belief is widespread that they *should* react negatively to their husband's use of these common words. To the wife with wholesome sexual attitudes, however, there is nothing offensive in the words he employs when he speaks to her of their sexual love; she doesn't find them "crude" or "dirty." His words tell her of his desires; with the same freedom, she expresses her sexual feelings. Both aid the sexual imagery of the other and hence increase their mutual arousal.

Touch: No one has ever adequately explained the pleasure we experience in physical contact with another. An infant stops crying when picked up by its mother. A sick child begs to have its forehead stroked. Lovers lose themselves in dreams as they hold hands. But what it is that gives us pleasure and expresses love in touching, and being touched, is a mystery—a very delightful mystery, however.

In marital relations, perhaps the major communication of emotions takes place on what might be called the "tactual level." It is through touch, and the caresses of love-making, that husband and wife are brought to the summit of arousal. While it would be difficult to overemphasize the importance of tactile stimulation in love-making, it might be equally difficult to exaggerate the problems which stem from a lack of understanding of it.

In order to give the fullest enjoyment to each other, husband and wife should attempt to learn something of the response of the opposite sex to caressing, and, what is more important, the desires and responses of the one to whom they are married. In this, men have more to learn than women. They must discover, most often by "trial and error," the caresses which will be most meaningful, loving, and most sexually stimulating. Many women are deprived of the full satisfaction of love-making through nothing more than ignorance on the part of their husbands. (Often, of course, as we mentioned before, they must accept a part of the blame for not making their desires known.)

Unlike a man's body, there are many areas of the female body which can properly be called sexual. Sexologists have found it convenient to divide these into *primary* and *secondary* erogenous areas. The primary erogenous areas are those which, when stimulated, will usually evoke the strongest sexual response. These include the nipples, the clitoris, and the vagina. The secondary areas, while less responsive to erotic stimulation, should not be thought of as less important. They literally extend over her entire body, and it is the hands of the lover caressing her body which release the deepest emotions within her. The secondary areas most frequently listed by women are the ears, throat, nape of the neck, breasts, small of the back, abdomen, buttocks, and inner thigh. But it is only her husband, motivated by love, who can discover the caresses which give her the greatest pleasure.

As she gains experience in love-making, she finds that these erogenous areas have a way of increasing in number as well as sensitivity such that more areas of her body become increasingly responsive to his touch. For his part, the husband learns not only the sensitive areas of her body, but the variety of caresses which will be most stimulating.

Love-making will usually progress from the secondary to the primary. But the loving caresses of husband and wife serve as far more than sexual stimuli in preliminary love-making. They communicate tenderness, warmth, support, and a host of other affections. And so, they become expressions of love many times other than when the couple are engaging in sexual love-making. This point may seem readily apparent, but more than a few husbands neglect physical signs of affection except when they desire sexual relations. It's little wonder that their wives so often feel unloved and bitter.

Touching and caressing the primary erogenous areas must be considered a major part of love-making. It brings her to the point of readiness for intercourse. And, more important, it is often directly related to the ultimate satisfaction a woman will derive from love-making. This is especially true of clitoral stimulation. Caressing of this small, highly sensitive, organ should usually be considered an essential part of pre-coital love-making. Like all love-making, this should never be done in a cursory way. His genital caresses should at all times communicate his love for her. Being so sensitive, the clitoris can be painfully irritated by stimulation if the husband's caresses are hurried and rough, rather than lovingly patient and tender. In developing this skill, the husband should take his cues from his wife, and she should feel free to express her feelings and desires.

It is usually accepted that men do not have secondary erogenous areas, at least not comparable to women. It would be a mistake, however, to conclude from this that a wife's caresses are not stimulating or pleasurable. Any loving physical contact between spouses can be exciting and sexually arousing. But most men are less sexually responsive than women to non-genital caresses.

The glans of the penis is, by far, the most sensitive to erotic stimulation. While tactile stimulation of other parts of the body, especially in the genital region, is usually arousing, it is the head of the penis, alone, which can properly be designated a primary erogenous area in the male. Although a husband's physical readiness for intercourse will usually not be dependent upon such stimulation, and hence it cannot be considered "essential" in the manner in which we spoke of caressing the clitoris, the loving wife, realizing the sensations it evokes and the pleasure it gives, will make it an "essential" part of her love-making. And since, as we pointed out, the reactions to our love-making, in a good marriage, are reciprocal, she will become increasingly aroused by touching him. Nevertheless, not all wives experience pleasure in caressing their husbands. Some even find it repugnant. But these wives would do well to recognize that these negative reactions are not those of a *woman* who has found the freedom of sexual love. And if she is motivated to love her husband, she will subject these attitudes to some self-searching evaluation.

Taste and *Smell:* Just as with the other senses, we might attempt to divide tastes and odors into primary and secondary sexual stimuli. Here, however, the division is not as apparent, and probably not as valid. For, while the savored glass of wine shared by the lovers and the fragrance of night-blooming jasmine in the bedroom may be considered secondary stimuli, there are no specific tastes or odors which can rightly be called primary sexual stimuli.

These romantic tastes and odors can make a delightful contribution to the love-making art, however. It may be the common association between taste and sexual arousal which accounts for so many foods at one period or another having been attributed with aphrodisiac properties. While no food or drink has been proven to be a sexual stimulant, eating and drinking together, especially in an appropriate setting, has to be classed as a romantic stimulus. But this may be carrying our designation a bit too far since we can't be sure what constitutes the romantic stimulus, the setting or the taste or both. This would also apply, for example, to the romantic value of roses; is it their color, texture, odor, or all of these? Not that it really matters. It's enough to recognize and accept romance and all that contributes to it; we don't need to analyze it.

We may not be able to speak of primary stimuli in this area, but some odors and tastes approach this degree of stimulation. The scent of the body in particular, can be a strong erotic stimulant and would come closest to meeting the definition. Both the scent and taste of the body were emphasized as sexual stimuli in what is surely the most moving profession of erotic love, the Song of Songs of King Solomon:

Sweet, sweet are your caresses, my bride, my true love; wine cannot ravish the senses like that embrace, nor any spices match the perfume that breathes from you. Sweet are your lips, my bride, as honey dripping from its comb; honey-sweet your tongue, and soft as milk; the perfume of your garments is very incense. My bride, my true love, a close garden; hedged all about, a spring shut in and sealed! What wealth of grace is here!

The lover doesn't speak here of the scent of artificial perfumes; he sings of "the perfume that breathes from you." Perfumes, subtly applied, blend with the natural scent of the body and act to enhance its fragrance, but it is the natural scent of the body which is, or should be, most stimulating. The cosmetic industries have amassed fortunes through persuading the public that body odor is offensive. But the natural odors of the body can be offensive only if the body is unclean, and it should be apparent that a concern for personal cleanliness is a testimony of love since in love-making they each present their body to the other.

Taste, as an erotic stimulus, is more difficult to define. There is little doubt that the taste of the skin and lips can be stimulating. But when the poet speaks of the "sweetness" of his lover's lips, it is to more than taste that he is responding. It is to a *kiss.*

Kissing holds a place of such importance in sexual

stimulation and the expression of love that it has come to symbolize erotic love. It truly deserves to be classed as a major source of sexual arousal.

Erotic stimulation of the lips and mouth—kissing—is usually the first shared sexual experience of a boy and girl. It is their introduction into a world of adult sexuality. Can anyone ever forget that first kiss? Or the feelings it aroused (although we may not have admitted it even to ourselves)? There can be little question that these feelings can be intense. So, when parents become concerned over adolescents engaging indiscriminately in prolonged kissing, they are speaking from a mature recognition of the powerful desires it can ignite.

Sexual love can vary greatly in its expression, but it would be difficult to picture the making of love which would not draw the couple to return, again and again, to the communion of the lover's kiss. The desire, submission, and commitment which they communicate in the touch of their lips give a continuing reassurance of love which permits the fullest sexual expression.

Various euphemisms have been employed in referring to the prolonged erotic kiss in which the tongues of the lovers meet and penetrate between each others' lips. Frequently, boys and girls of dating age are warned of the moral danger in "soul kissing." Often, this is merely another undefined label. They may also hear it called "french" kissing. But these words may have no meaning until they are introduced to the practice—sometimes only to find it a disturbing experience. This is particularly so if the girl (or boy) has been raised in a rigid, anti-sexual environment. One young bride told us she was shocked when her husband attempted such a kiss; her mother had told her the practice was perverted! If the attitudes of husband and wife are wholesome, however, they can be expected to find marital kissing a tender expression of love.

It isn't difficult to understand why such deep kissing is so extremely stimulating. The tongue penetrating between the other's lips is homologous to the penetration of the sexual union. Little wonder then that it is such a natural part of love-making; it anticipates, and promises, the complete union which will follow.

It might be more accurate to talk of marital kisses, *plural.* The prolonged deep kissing of the lips is but one, of several, marital kisses. The kissing of any part of the body can be highly arousing to both partners. A husband's tender kisses on the throat and fingertips, while not, perhaps, intrinsically erotic, may add greatly to his wife's total sexual response. Hence, they can be considered at least secondary stimuli. And the same is true, of course, of her kisses. "Covering each other with kisses" should be more than a poetic expression.

There are other kisses which are primary sexual stimuli. Kissing the breasts, particularly the nipples, and stimulating the nipples with the lips and tongue must be classed with these. As a primary erogenous area, the nipples rank second only to the clitoris in erotic sensitivity. Some women, in fact, are able to achieve orgasm through nothing more than stimulation of their nipples. With most couples, kissing and caressing the breasts is an abiding source of excitement and pleasure, one which they enjoy throughout love-making. Many wives enjoy having their breasts caressed and their nipples stimulated for long periods of time. A husband should keep in mind, however, that a woman's breasts, and particularly the nipples, are very sensitive and easily irritated or bruised. Any rough handling of her breasts, therefore, could be very painful, and might even result in injury.

The most stimulating marital kiss, for both sexes, involves the oral stimulation of the genitals. It is also the most misunderstood and therefore, the most potentially troublesome. In spite of the increasing candor with which sexuality is discussed, oral-genital acts are deleted from many essays on marital sexuality. By impliedly treating the subject as taboo, however, the writers have left many young couples, striving to grow in marital love, to conclude that these acts are unnatural and immoral. A bride in her twenties told of separating from her husband because he suggested it. She said she loved him, but she felt sure her love wasn't returned. "How could he love me, and ask me to do something degrading and sinful?" Unfortunately, she had never discussed it with her confessor; it was "too disgusting to even talk about." Had she done so, she might have spared herself many tearful nights.

Stimulation of the penis by the lips and tongue is called *fellatio.* Oral stimulation of the clitoris is called *cunnilingus.* While this form of pre-coital love-making is engaged in by many, perhaps most, married couples, the apparent prohibition against discussion of it has led more than a few to conclude that they were virtually alone in the practice of a "depravity." Such is not the case. Psychiatrists and psychologists can point to a number of studies verifying the prevalence of this variety of love-making among married couples. Of course, the acceptance of a practice, no matter how widespread, can never be employed as a criterion of morality, nor as an argument to condone an immoral act. But here, this isn't an issue. Oral-genital stimulation *in the pre-coital love-making of husband and wife* is not immoral. Nor is it unnatural or perverted.

But we have tried to describe marital sexuality in terms of beauty and love. What about oral-genital sexuality? Recently, this question was raised at a pre-marital discussion we addressed. A young woman pointed out that we had described sexual love with beauty; but would this also apply to these actions? We told her we felt it did. If husband and wife have found love in their sexual union and the freedom which accompanies it, they will find it not only extremely arousing, but beautiful.

Occasionally, we hear husbands or wives who object to the practice on the grounds that the genitals are "unclean" and genital kissing is unhygienic. As many authorities have pointed out, however, where personal cleanliness is a part of the preparation for love-making, as it should be, there is nothing unclean about the genital organs. Usually this view stems from an unfortunate early association between things sexual and "dirtiness," an association the couple would do well to discard.

If there is a single point which should be emphasized, it is that love-making should always be directed toward making love in all the ways that will give the most to the loved one. It should never be hurried, never a "means to an end." Husbands, especially, often need to be reminded of this; too many wives justifiably complain of being hurried in love-making by husbands who seem always in a rush to complete the act. No art can be rushed if it is to retain its quality as art; and only if it retains an element of time-lessness, can the love-making become an artistic creation of beauty. It must be approached with patience, imagination, and the desire to create a sexual union that will reflect the awesome mystery of the vocation to which husband and wife are called. Only then can it become an art, and only then can it become fully loving.

Sexual love is always an adventure—a very beautiful and exciting adventure. It is the adventure of one man and one woman, both seeking through love to become *one* in their marriage. It can never be the same for any two couples; and for each couple the expressions of love will be as constantly varying as the colors of a kaleidoscope. We have tried only to point to some of the multicolored pieces which form and re-form in these ever-changing patterns, and, hopefully, to add a few pieces that may have been overlooked.

It is the sunlight shining through and reflecting the pieces, bits of colored glass and amber, which gives the pattern in the kaleidoscope its beauty. Through the bits and pieces of their love-making, the couple see deep within each other to glimpse the beauty reflected by the light of their sacramental love.

CHAPTER VIII

Coitus

THROUGH THE INITIAL sexual union, the marriage is consummated. It comes into full existence and is stamped with indissolubility. In joining their bodies, man and wife very literally unite "in one flesh." Only a mother and her unborn child could be more so.

Love is the seeking to be united, to become *one*, with another. In the marital union, it reaches its highest human fulfillment. The painful separateness which is the longing for love vanishes in an act which is physical, psychological, and spiritual. He gives his body to her, places his seed within her, and, in total surrender, she receives him. And in accepting him, not in a mere physical compliance, but in the selflessness of love, she gives herself. In faith, she entrusts her future to him. In hope, she seeks fulfillment in him. In love, she finds God—with him.

Most simply described, coitus is the introduction of the penis into the vagina, followed by ejaculation. But in speaking of marriage, even on a physical level, this description is inadequate. In humans, the sexual union is an act of love, not a mere act of mating. If we think of it only in terms of such literalism, it is devoid of love and stripped of its human quality. This, tragically, is what much of our society tends to do.

We have said, and we repeat, that love-making cannot properly be thought of in terms of stages. It builds in a crescendo of desire toward its consummation. The mutual arousal of the couple makes this a very natural transition. Their arousal, nurtured by physical expressions of love, leads them to the marital embrace, not in a compulsion, nor a demand, but in a desire to complete the giving of self.

But these desires must be communicated. How else are they each to know? She must "tell" him, verbally or otherwise, that she is physically ready, and desires, to receive him. It is the only means by which he can know; the only way in which he can meet her needs. Marital love, even when it approaches its fullest growth, does not endow the couple with an ability to read minds. He cannot *see* her thoughts and feelings; only she can know them fully. Since she alone is aware of her state of arousal, it is her responsibility to signal her readiness; and his, to await her signal. By patiently leading her to the point where she eagerly seeks to accept his body, he increases his own satisfaction, insures her sexual fulfillment, and furthers the transcendence of their marital union. For this to succeed, communication between the spouses is imperative.

Husband and wife may communicate their feelings and desires on a variety of levels, directly or indirectly, verbally or nonverbally. With the growth of their marriage, the couple develop a system which is theirs alone. It is their "language of love." Through it, they express their love for each other; and through it, they each learn the ways to best love the other. So long as the language is clearly understood by both, it makes little difference how the "messages" are conveyed. Words, gestures, even facial expressions may suffice. The important issue is not *how* they communicate, but *how well*. Communication, however, is rarely developed sufficiently to rely upon the subtlety of a fleeting glance. Vague and ambiguous messages can give rise to misunderstandings; and misunderstandings can leave scars. Words, plain and unambiguous, are still the best means of communication. This is especially true in the expression of sexual desires and feelings. Both husband and wife should work to develop within themselves the *freedom* to do so. Together, they should strive to develop a *method* of doing so.

The initial experience of the marital embrace should be the commencement of a lifelong vocation of love. It should be an occasion of joy and an experience of beauty. Why then, do so many make it sound like an ordeal? Why is it that frequently we hear it discussed solely in terms of a "loss of virginity"? There are scores of marriage books in which the emphasis is on rupturing of the hymen. And too often, the description given of this event is frightening, or disgusting, or both. Having read such material, a young bride may approach the consummation of her marriage in terror. The young husband may also be apprehensive and reluctant to subject his wife to such a "traumatic ordeal." It would be difficult to overestimate the negative effect of such writings. They transform the marital bed into a chamber of horrors.

Virginity is not something which is "lost." Virginity is the *state* of being a virgin, of not having experienced sexual relations. It is a negative, rather than positive, condition. Negative in the sense that it is the non-occurrence of an event. It is the consummation of the marriage in sexual intercourse which is a positive experience. It is a mutual offering which deepens the meaning of the marital commitment and bestows grace. It is a gift which they each receive, not a treasure which they lose. Furthermore, love is that which we *give*, not that which we *give up!*

Recently, in discussing with parents some of the issues raised during a series of talks to high school students, a mother of four girls said, "Well, I hope that you stressed what I tell my daughters, that the most important gift they can give their husbands is their virginity." No, we didn't. Nor do we agree. It seems to us that this presents a view which distorts the virtue of chastity. It may, furthermore, be seriously misleading, even harmful.

Practice of the virtue of chastity, prior to marriage, demands celibacy. It is a moral law, based upon the divinely ordained use of the sexual faculty. We accept it and keep it out of love for God, not out of desire to please a future spouse. In the sacrament of Matrimony, we each give ourself completely to the person to whom we are joined. And it is with, and through, that person that we give ourself to God. From Him, we receive the joys and graces of our vocation—not the least of which is the profound benediction of the marital union.

The attitude toward virginity which makes it a "gift" which the bride presents to her husband, and which stresses its loss in the marital consummation can only harm a marriage. It may, to some extent, stem from a faulty concept of *consecrated virginity,* a term used to refer to the celebate state of the religious. The words, *consecrated virginity,* however, are ambiguous. The "calling" in a religious vocation (including the vocation of Christian marriage) is to the service of God. And the commitment which is made in answer to the vocation is to Him. To interpret this, and emphasize it, as a commitment to celibacy, rather than to God, is to demean the vocation. Furthermore, it tends rather egocentrically to focus on the sacrifice the individual offers *to* God rather than on the privilege offered the individual *by* God. Virginity, we must understand, is not, per se, a virtue; chastity is a virtue. And yet how often the virtue of chastity is implicitly defined as celibacy. Even some writers who should know better fall into this error. If we make this mistake, the marital union may be construed as a fall from virtue (but one which is somehow condoned). Those responsible for pre-marital counseling might do well to impress upon the bride-to-be the sanctifying character of the marital union, to point out to her that when she gives herself to her husband in the consummation of their marriage, she is giving herself not only in justice and love, but also in chastity.

Those who picture the consummation of the marriage as an act of sacrifice rob many young women of the joy which should accompany the introduction to marital love. While most brides recall their wedding night as a tender and beautiful experience, there are others who remember it as a nightmare of pain, disgust, and bitterness. The latter reaction, however, is seldom related to any physical difficulties, at least not in an anatomically functional sense. The problems are psychological rather than physical. Nevertheless, the emotional reactions can affect and interact with the physical, and the result may leave memories which cut deeply and leave lasting scars. Unwholesome attitudes and unfounded fears often combine to set the stage for such reactions. If then, in addition, the husband is insensitive or callous in his approach, the experience may result in loathing rather than loving.

Such tragedies need not occur. With proper instruction, wholesome attitudes, and with a patience and tenderness motivated by loving concern for each other, the initial sexual union will be a pleasurable, and beautifully memorable, experience for both.

The marital union may be satisfactorily completed in any of several postural positions. Some marriage manuals devote page after page to detailed description of allegedly different positions. Essentially, however, the nature of the act and the mechanics of the body, permit only a few basic variations. And certainly the desire to love should lead the couple to explore the means to best communicate their love; detailed word blueprints should hardly be necessary.

These postural differences, however, can play an important role in the love-making. Like all else, they touch on the psychological as well as the physical dimensions of the relationship. A preference for one or another position, just as with other preferences in love-making, often has "meaning" and communicates emotional needs, although neither spouse may be conscious of such needs.

There is no one "normal" position for sexual intercourse. Any posture the couple assume, standing, sitting, or reclining, in which the sexual union can be completed, is "normal." We can only speak of *the* normal position if we are thinking in terms of a "norm," that is, one which is most frequently employed. But this, as some investigators have discovered, is at least somewhat determined by the culture. What is usually referred to as the "normal" coital position in our culture is infrequently employed in some non-Western cultures. In this position, the wife lies prone, on her back; the husband lies in a face-to-face position on top of her. To both husband and wife, this usually seems a very "natural" position. Permitting, as it does, physical contact over the length of their bodies, bringing their faces close together, it increases the physical intimacy reflective of the emotional and spiritual unity toward which they strive. Nevertheless, it is but one of several possible positions. What is important is the preference of the couple, and the freedom from unhealthy emotional and moral blocks which permit them to make a choice. Probably their preferences will vary from time to time; certainly the emotional needs and desires of husband and wife are never static.

The "naturalness" of the face-to-face position leads some to mistakenly conclude that other coital positions are "unnatural"—and, hence, immoral. The notion is absurd.

Furthermore, it may be destructive. It may inhibit, rather than enhance, the free expression of marital love. To assert the morality of only a single position for marital relations is as fallacious as would be the contention that there is only one propitious way to say "I love you."

The various positions for intercourse may be classified in several ways: face-to-face positions, positions where both face the same direction, positions in which the husband is the active partner, positions in which the wife is the active partner, etc. In addition to the so-called normal position, the couple may engage in intercourse face-to-face lying on their sides, or by the husband lying prone on his back and his wife lying on top, or by the husband lying prone on his back and the wife sitting astride him. They may complete the act facing in the same direction, the husband approaching above and behind her. In this position, she may be lying prone or kneeling in a knee-chest position. They may further vary the act by assuming sitting or standing positions. Only the imagination of the couple and/or their inhibitions will curtail "experimenting" to discover variations in love-making.

The unmarried or newly wed might ask, "Why try different positions?" For the happily married, the answer is never that love-making in a single position has become dull or monotonous. The reason is first of all that the different positions convey differing emotions and meet differing psychological needs, although these may be subtle and the couple may not be aware that these motivate their choices. But there is also a more obvious reason. In changing positions, they change the angle of insertion of the penis and the depth of penetration; this, of course, will vary the areas of greatest stimulation, and, since their physical as well as psychological needs fluctuate, the sensations may be more intense and pleasurable in one position at one time and in another position the next.

One point should be kept in mind: the position, emotionally and philosophically, that the couple maintain *toward* the sexual union is far more important than the physical positions they select *for* the act.

Love-making, especially coitus, has a tempo, an ever-changing tempo. It will fluctuate, increase and decrease, throughout the love-making. Somewhat, this will reflect the increasing pleasure and arousal of both husband and wife. It will also contribute to their arousal. Thus, the tempo of love-making contributes to arousal, and the increased arousal state affects, in turn, the tempo. But, while sexual arousal usually increases, almost monotonically, to the point of climax, the tempo may, at times, be intentionally slowed by either spouse. In learning to do so, they prolong their mutual enjoyment, and increase their ultimate satisfaction. There is another, more important, reason, however. Following orgasm, it is usually difficult for a man to continue the movements of coitus. Usually he will feel physically expended, but, more important, in most men the glans becomes almost painfully sensitive to further stimulation, and they find it virtually impossible to continue coital movements after ejaculation. Hence, if the wife has not yet achieved orgasm, she may remain sexually unfulfilled. It may leave her tense and restless, or even irritable. Should it occur frequently, and with little or no concern evidenced by the husband, she may grow resentful of what appears to be his exploitive approach to the marital union. In any case, marital relations in which only one of the spouses regularly achieves full satisfaction can never serve to unify, only divide.

It is usually the husband, acting on cues from his wife, who directs the tempo. He strives to give the fullest expression of love, and the greatest sexual pleasure, to her. Since, however, with tactual stimulation, the male orgasm is usually more quickly reached, he will frequently find it necessary to slow the tempo in order to insure her satisfaction.

The wife, may, of course, reach orgasm before her husband but, unlike a man, a woman ordinarily does not then find it difficult to continue coitus until his orgasm is achieved, especially if she is permitted a short respite following climax. It is not at all unusual for a sexually mature (and happily married) woman to experience orgasm two, three, or even several times during the course of the love-making. The orgasms may occur prior to, as well as during, the marital union.

Experiencing multiple orgasm during marital love is not in any way abnormal. It is no indication that a woman is "over-sexed," "animalistic," or "unwomanly," as some wives have confessed to feeling. Nor should a wife have any fears that it is a violation of marital chastity. It is not. Attaining orgasm once or several times is a matter of temperament, sexual maturity, preferences, and the love-making art of the couple. With many, this will vary from time to time, as will most all other dimensions of sexual love.

The answer, as always, must be found in loving. It is in and through loving that the meaning of orgasm is found. Position, tempo, multiple orgasm, and all of the diverse and complex sexual actions and reactions are, in themselves, of little importance—so long as both spouses hold a strong desire to love. Their love will transcend the overconcern for these strictly physical parameters which plague so many couples. Without it, the act is a thing apart, a dehumanized encounter that no degree of sexual skills and techniques can make whole. To set the attainment of orgasm, per se, as the goal of sexual love, is to miss the essential meaning of the marital union. Furthermore, such a goal-oriented physical approach can be expected to deter, rather than aid, the mutual growth in sexual love so necessary to a Christian marriage.

Following the sexual climax, there is a great release of tension. It brings with it a feeling of relaxation and tranquillity. The anxieties and frustrations which are so much a part of human existence seem, at least for a time, to fade. There is less obsession with *things,* less compulsion to be *doing,* more acceptance of, and satisfaction in, *being.* There is a timelessness accompanying the unity which is felt. It should be a time during which the world is shut out, during which their love deepens, nurtured by their closeness and the joy they have found in the gift each has given and received.

Frequently, however, we talk to couples, one or both of whom neglect this post-coital period of love. In the majority of these cases, the husband is to blame. Many wives complain that their husbands abruptly cease making love and virtually ignore them as soon as the act is completed. The husband's actions may, of course, be wholly egocentric. On the other hand, there are many husbands who do not lack regard for their wives, but rather lack knowledge of feminine sexuality.

Following orgasm, a man will ordinarily experience a feeling of satiation and exhaustion. From the emotional peak at the moment of ejaculation, male excitation drops sharply. Many husbands, almost at once, desire sleep. Women, however, approach the sexual climax in a more gradual manner. And, following orgasm, female excitation diminishes in a similarly gradual fashion; there is not the abrupt decline characteristic of the male. The wife's desire for sexual love is not extinguished with orgasm. It is not the sharp peak followed by a sudden drop, but rather a summit on which she finds a plateau. As long as she can, she attempts to linger there, savoring its awesome beauty. Only reluctantly does she descend. Her need for physical love remains strong at that time; it only changes in character. It is a need to be held by him, to feel his support and strength, to cling to the closeness of the moment, to be reassured, through words and caresses, of his love for her.

Should he, whether through lack of understanding or lack of loving, sharply end the love-making and draw back from her embrace, the timelessness of the moment will be shattered and the afterglow of their sexual love will be extinguished. This should be a period of closeness, a period of true communion, a period during which husband and wife pledge their love by touch and by word. It should be a period of renewal, of hope, and of joy.

CHAPTER IX

Love-making: Psychological Aspects

ADAM GREETED EVE as "bone of my bone, and flesh of my flesh." Plato told the story of the androgyne, the myth that man was originally both male and female but, as punishment for having offended the gods, was split in two and male and female separated; human love, then, is the striving to restore this lost unity. Both stories give recognition to a significant psychological truth: man and woman are two halves of a whole; they are completed only through each other. The sexual union is the psychophysical expression of this seeking for completeness. In each act of sexual love, we strive to find a psychological unity through physically becoming *one*.

There is still much to be discovered about the nature of man and the nature of woman; we have really only scratched the surface. Much of the time we tend to overlook the very important fact that the sexes are complementary rather than opposite, that they need each other, and that any denial of this need can only hinder emotional growth. In fact, if the sexes were truly "opposite" there could be virtually no meaningful human interaction between them. They would come in contact only to exploit and be exploited. Even on a biological level, the sexes are not really opposite. Both carry the hormone of the other sex as well as their own. Both have traits and personality characteristics "typical" of the other. Sexually, both are active as well as passive; both are dominant as well as submissive. Their personality dimensions are measurable in *degree* rather than in *kind*.

But there are differences between the sexes, very important ones. And these essential differences between masculine and feminine psychology evidence themselves in no area of human existence more than in the sexual union.

While conceding that we are on less than firm ground whenever we attempt to differentiate the emotional characteristics of the sexes, some differences are, nevertheless, so universally observable that we are probably safe in assuming that they are rooted deep in the psychobiology of male and female. As a starting point, however, it might be best to sketch briefly the sequence of steps in the psychosexual development of a child without attempting to separate that which is innate from that which is culturally imposed, and without trying to analyze differing effects as a function of sexual differences. All, obviously, are major determinants of behavior, but it would seem of little value to try to find a psychological midpoint between the extremes of Freud ("anatomy is a woman's destiny") and Simone de Beauvoir ("one is not born, but becomes a woman").

We will employ Freudian theory as our framework, not because we are "Freudian" (we are not), nor because the validity of the theory has been established, but because empirical observation has shown the theory to be the most useful in understanding the development of the child and, more importantly, the most valuable in predicting adult sexual behavior.

In Freudian theory, the *libido* is the *drive*, the motivating, or life, force. It motivates the individual to seek pleasure and avoid pain. While primarily sexual in nature, it includes much more than the strictly sexual. All desire for human contact has its origin in this drive force. It is the libido, from infancy on, which motivates the individual to progress through the various psychosexual stages toward mature adult heterosexuality. If the environment, and primarily the parental relationship, is emotionally healthy, this is a fairly orderly progression. If, on the other hand, the child encounters major emotional obstacles, the libido may become "fixated" at any of these stages prior to maturity. This fixation will then show itself in emotional problems throughout adolescence and continue on in adulthood.

One of the few truly innate behaviors that we note in the newborn child is the sucking instinct. If its cheek is lightly stroked, the infant will begin to make sucking movements. During the first year of life, the libidinal energy is centered in the mouth. All gratification is derived orally. The baby's life is little more than a cycle of eating and sleeping. This is the *oral* stage of psychosexual development. The *sexual* aspects in this and the following stage may not be readily apparent. In fact, at the time Freud introduced the theory, many people were outraged. To suggest the notion of infantile sexuality in the Victorian culture of Vienna at the turn of the century was unspeakably offensive. Even today, many find it difficult to accept. They seem to feel it impugns the innocence of childhood. A residual of the oral stage, however, is easily observed as a component of adult sexual behavior, as well as many less overtly sexual gratifications. Kissing, oral stimulation of the breasts, and oral-genital acts are rather obvious examples.

Freud called the next stage, the period from about ages one to three, the *anal* stage. This is usually the period of toilet training, an activity which, unless it is approached with good sense, can be a frustrating experience for both parent and child. During this stage, the child discovers pleasure can be derived from the retention and expulsion of feces, and that reward and punishment can attach to this bodily function. The child's interests during this time are largely self-centered; the child seeks gratification from its own body and its functions. It is a narcissistic period, the residuals of which can be seen in the egocentric approach to human relationships of some adults. Fixation can occur during this period also if the emotional climate of the home is unhealthy. The direct relationship to adult sexuality of the *anal* stage is not so obvious, but it is nonetheless real.

Following the anal period, at about age three, the child enters the final pregenital phase of development, the *phallic* stage. The libido becomes centered in the genital organs, the penis in the boy and the clitoris in the girl. The child discovers the pleasurable sensations experienced in self-stimulation. It is a very natural period of exploration. Unfortunately, some parents become unduly concerned when they discover the child playing with his or her genitals and make an "issue" of what is normal behavior at this age. In doing so, they may sow seeds of guilt and fear which will prove difficult to uproot.

One of the written questions submitted following a recent talk typified the view of far too many parents: "How do you handle the problem of a four-year-old boy innocently handling his penis?" The question would seem to answer itself. If the action is *innocent*—and it most certainly cannot be otherwise—where does the "problem" lie, with the child or with the parent? The "problem" will not become a "problem" unless we, as parents, make it so. At that age, we might better ignore it, and accept it as a normal part of development, or we may find that we have created a real problem, one that may affect the child from then on.

Soon, the child enters the most important period in the psychosexual development, the *Oedipal* period. This period, which usually extends from about ages three to seven, is part of the phallic stage and is the initial introduction to inter-personal affective relationships. Freud took the name from the Greek drama, *Oedipus Rex*. In this ancient legend, Oedipus unknowingly kills his father and takes his mother as his wife. When he later learns the true identity of the woman he has married, he blinds himself in an act of remorse and self-hatred. During the Oedipal period, the child directs its emotional (sexual) interests, toward the parent of the opposite sex and develops feelings of rivalry toward the parent of the same sex. This, admittedly, is not an easy theory for many to accept. When Freud first hypothesized the Oedipus complex, even a number of his colleagues were less than accepting. After all, it did seem to be accusing a child of incestuous desires! What Freud was theorizing, however, was not a dark perversion, but a normal stage of development through which the child experiences its first heterosexual response. Obviously, this is not the conscious, overt, sexual reaction we experience as adults, but any perceptive parent has observed the "attachment" the child shows during this period to the parent of the opposite sex. This is the pre-school age during which the daughter becomes "daddy's girl" and the son becomes "mommie's little man."

This period can be one of great conflict and anxiety for the child. If the relationship between the parents is wholesome, that is, if there is a mature love between them, the parent-child relationships may be expected to be healthy and the conflict will be successfully resolved and a healthy personality will develop in the child. If these interactions have been traumatic, however, the libido will remain fixated at the Oedipal level and serious psycho-sexual problems will result. Residuals of the Oedipal stage may affect the choice of a spouse and the manner in which husband and wife interact. And it may profoundly affect their sexual relations, often adversely.

From about age seven until the onset of puberty, the child goes through a period of relative sexual quiescence. This is the phase of life Freud designated as the *latency* period. During this period, there is little attraction to the opposite sex; boys prefer to play with boys, and girls want little to do with boys. There is sexual curiosity and activity during this period, but for the most part, it is an interim period.

With the onset of puberty, all this changes. There is an increased sexual awareness accompanying the many physical changes. Suddenly the world and all those in it seems changed. This awareness brings a reactivation of the Oedipal feelings. If the original Oedipal conflict has been resolved with relative success, the adolescent is able to transfer his or her sexual interest to members of the other sex outside the family. At this point, the libido enters the final stage leading to mature sexuality, the *genital* stage. Each of these stages of development present their own problems. In a healthy emotional environment the child passes from one to the next with little difficulty and reaches the goal of adulthood with normal heterosexual feelings. A variety of circumstances may, of course, exist during childhood which will disrupt the normal development, most of them, according to Freud, resulting in unresolved Oedipal conflicts. It would be unrealistic to attempt to even briefly describe the psychosexual problems which may result. To one degree or another, impotency, prema-ture ejaculation, frigidity, and a host of other problems may be rooted in unresolved Oedipal attachments. It may not be the "singular cause" as Freud implies, but it does exist as a powerful influence, one which undermines many marriages.

Freud described infantile sexuality as "polymorphous perverse." The words are unfortunate, conveying, as they do, a pejorative significance. But this was not Freud's intent. As he employed the words, they described what he believed to be the normal direction of the sexual instinct in the child. In the infant, Freud said, there is no determined sexual object or form of expression. It merely seeks its own satisfaction. As the child matures, social influences, particularly the parents, direct the child's sexual interests toward a particular object, ordinarily the other sex. But originally, the sexual instinct is undifferentiated with regard to its object and its goal.

Actually, there is little evidence to support this portion of Freud's theory. In some respects, it is even inconsistent with other parts of his theory. Nearly all observation would seem to refute any hypothesis of an undifferentiated sexual instinct. We hardly need cite empirical evidence to support the view that man and woman are, by nature, attracted to each other. Nevertheless, there is something to be learned from Freud's observations of the "polymorphous perverse." It can be directed toward sexual objects and goals other than normal heterosexuality. This much we know. But we need also to understand that there is a polymorphous aspect to normal adult sexuality. And that this is in no way perversion. What we mean is that normal sexuality, while heterosexual, and directed toward the goal of coitus, is widely varied, and that the normal adult is, at least in some degree, responsive to a broad spectrum of sexual stimuli.

Many of the varied aspects of sexual love we have discussed in the last two chapters reflect the normal polymorphous sexual interest of man and woman. Unless we understand what is "normal," however, we may observe the obvious similarities between these variations in love-making and certain abnormal sexual practices, and mistakenly conclude that these normal practices are perverse. In normal mature sexuality, the sexual "object" is another adult of the opposite sex; the sexual "goal" is coitus. In sexual perversion, the individual's sexual interests become centered in a different object or goal. Unless this distinction is clear, a couple may either restrict the expression of their sexual love out of fear that their desires may be "abnormal" or may suffer unnecessary guilt. To illustrate this distinction, let's take the case of voyeurism. The normal man finds sexual enjoyment, and arousal, in looking at the female body. If a man doesn't, in fact, find such viewing pleasurable, we might suspect some psychosexual problem. The sexual arousal that results will then center on the sexual object, a woman, and be directed toward the goal of sexual intercourse. In the sexual deviation of voyeurism, on the other hand, the goal is the voyeuristic act itself; satisfaction is achieved through the *looking*.

With the popularizing of Freudian theory, it was perhaps inevitable that some individuals would use Freudian theory to try to find symptoms in every action and would "interpret" and "analyze" all human signs of affection in terms of "fixations" and "complexes." In some circles, this has become a sort of cocktail party pastime, but a not too kind one. Not only are these interpretations generally incorrect, they are often made with a lack of charity which borders on viciousness. In nearly every case, they imply that this or that sexual preference, interest, or behavior indicates some sort of repressed abnormal desire. Should a man show an interest in large-bosomed women, these amateur "analysts" will be quick to point out his "oral fixation" and his unconscious desire for a nurturant "mother figure." Or if a young woman remarks on the attractiveness of a man with graying sideburns, she is accused of having an unhealthy attachment to her father. Virtually everything is given significance as a symbol or a symptom in this game. Unquestionably, many of our sexual preferences and associations are learned and may be traced to early experiences, but to find pathological significance in all sexual desires and actions is as potentially destructive as it is absurd. We can easily find oral, anal, narcissistic, sadomasochistic, Oedipal, and a wide range of other components in the total sexual behavior of normal adults. Furthermore, the stimuli which may elicit a sexual response, as we have indicated, can be infinitely varied. This is not only normal but uniquely human. It is one of the aspects which distinguishes the sexual union of man and woman from the copulation of lower animals. Even in the more intelligent animals, the sexual act follows an instinctual pattern; it is a mating act with little variety. Only in man does it take on the variation which gives it the mystery of romance; only in man does it reach maturity through a complex interaction of biological development and learned associations; and therefore, only in man can it be an act of *love*.

Psychologically, men are generally more dominant, analytic, extroverted, and aggressive than women. Women, on the other hand, are inclined to be more passive, intuitive, and introverted. These personality characteristics are important in any acts of sexual love, expressing, as they do, the total personalities of the partners. Some acts are clearly dominant, others submissive. The making of sexual love, however, involves a number of acts, not just one, and they may each express different facets of the personality, and differing, changing, emotional needs. Furthermore, these needs change from day to day, or even hour to hour, and from one period of love-making to the next.

With most couples, the male sexual role is *relatively* more aggressive and the female sexual role is *relatively* more passive, but throughout the love-making there are usually a number of "role reversals." We often tend to view the various acts of love-making in terms of masculine and feminine roles, and yet if the husband's actions were solely masculine (as it is usually defined), and the wife's role was entirely feminine, their sexual relations would be not only boring but brutal; it would be nothing more than the payment of the marital *debt*, in the worst possible meaning of the word!

We would be foolish to overly stress the psychological significance of the various acts of sexual love. If the couple have attained a degree of sexual maturity, they will play many and varied roles in their love-making. Their pre-coital love-making will not be constricted by questions of what is "masculine" or "feminine," nor will either of them feel their sexual identity is in any way threatened by this or that action or position for intercourse. In certain positions, such as with the woman astride, the wife's role is more active, but certainly no less feminine. Nor is a wife any less feminine if she, rather than her husband, initiates the love-making. It is neither a strictly masculine nor feminine role. As we mentioned previously, the husband is most often the wooer, but the wife who "seduces" her husband is expressing the best of her femininity.

When one of the partners insists upon one or another act or position to the exclusion of all others, however, it may indicate immature or unhealthy emotional needs, and may become a source of estrangement. A twenty-seven-year-old attorney, married six years, could enjoy marital relations only if his wife assumed the active role and permitted him to remain almost totally "passive." Seldom would he initiate the love-making; instead, he expected her to aggressively make all sexual overtures. The few times he had acceded to his wife's wishes and assumed the active role, he found himself unable to complete the act. His childhood training and experiences had bordered on the bizarre, and could be predicted to result in severe emotional difficulties, but be that as it may, it is obvious that his symptoms point to a serious psychosexual disturbance and not merely a sexual preference. Such cases are, fortunately, the exception. The actions or preferences become psychologically "significant" in such cases not because of their nature, nor because of a reversal in roles, but because of their exclusiveness.

Some couples find variety the spice of their love-making. Others, just as *normal*, find complete satisfaction year after year with little or no "experimentation." It only takes on importance if the couple are unable, because of fears, irrational inhibitions, or unhealthy sexual needs to introduce variety into their love-making.

Sexual climax in a man differs very significantly from climax in a woman. What he experiences should be representative of his total manhood; in her orgasm should be found the essence of her womanhood. We previously mentioned the controversy over the nature of the female orgasm. The issue is not a new one, and it hasn't lacked attention in books and journals. Very little, on the other hand, has been written about the male orgasm, and most of what has been written has been strictly physiological rather than psychological. But the psychological factors are as important in the male climax as they are in the female.

As the male approaches orgasm, his actions become increasingly aggressive and imperious. Physically, as well as psychologically, his sexual advances gradually change from persuasive and seductive to possessive and vanquishing: he *takes* her in the culmination of their love-making. This has often been likened to a combat which ends in a conquest. The nature of the act makes this a rather apparent analogy; there is always an element of conquest and submission in love-making, but the analogy is limited. He feels a strong desire to dominate, to bring her to the point of submission. He experiences pleasurable feelings of strength and power as he feels her surrender to him. At the moment of climax, his overwhelming desire is to enter her to the fullest. So, as the tempo of coitus increases and approaches ejaculation, his thrusts become more aggressive, and the depth of his insertion greater, so that when he achieves orgasm, it will ordinarily occur with the penis inserted as far as he is able. Although under at least a degree of conscious control, this deep thrust can be considered almost reflexive. On a biologic level, it serves an obvious purpose: the seminal fluid is ejaculated high in the vagina, thus aiding the sperm in its journey to impregnate the ovum. Psychologically, it is of such importance to sexual fulfillment in the man (and, for that matter, in the woman) that Freud at one time considered the contraceptive method of withdrawal at the point of orgasm (*coitus interruptus*) a causative factor in neurosis. (Thus, Freud sided with the moral theologians in condemning the practice, although admittedly for different reasons.)

We said the analogy was limited. The male actions, while aggressive and dominating, contain no element of hostility (unless we are speaking of rape rather than love). Therefore, the masculine "conquest" and the feminine "submission" resemble only superficially an engagement in battle. We might describe it paradoxically as a "loving combat." Man and woman play out the roles of their sexual natures. His desire to take and possess her is matched by her desire to surrender and be possessed. This is not apart from love; it is the basic nature of sexual love.

The desire to "conquer" which is so much a part of masculine sexuality, can easily be misinterpreted by the wife. Unless she has an understanding of male psychology, she may resent the imperiousness of his sexual behavior;

it may appear to be directed solely toward self-gratification. This is seldom so, however, even with the most selfish, unloving, husbands. The male ego, if nothing else, makes such behavior a rarity. Sexual adequacy is a very important component of the male self-image. Virtually every man wants to see himself as a "great lover." Hence, if a wife is not receiving sexual satisfaction, it may be more emotionally devastating to her husband than to herself. We have spoken to more than a few husbands who lost nearly all interest in marital relations when they found they were unable to give such satisfaction. For this reason, if no other, frigidity is as much a problem of the husband as the wife. In "conquering" her, he seeks a conquest of sexual love, one in which she surrenders herself to him in complete sexual fulfillment. If this doesn't result, he may see himself as a failure.

Something else makes the analogy less than perfect. Her surrender is in no way a vanquishment. Quite the contrary. If she feels that she must give in to her husband, surrender will be impossible; so will sexual satisfaction. Here we come up against an even greater paradox: the female orgasm.

A magazine arrived in today's mail carrying an article critical of what the authors see as an overemphasis on the quality of the female orgasm. They may have a valid point. There is, to be sure, a great deal of nonsense written about it. Much of it emphasizes the mechanics of sexual intercourse. They would have the reader believe that orgasm in a woman is solely related to physical techniques, and that the only thing of importance is the achievement of some sort of ecstatic sensation. In one such book, the female readers are instructed in exercises for the development of the vaginal muscles as the key to sexual bliss! So far, we haven't come across anything which tops that for absurdity! But to underscore the importance of the orgasm, as many psychotherapists have done, is not without merit. What makes it so important, however, is not just the question of whether a wife may or may not be experiencing a particular type of pleasure, no matter how great it may be, but rather what this may indicate about her whole personality and what she may or may not be as a woman.

Despite the position of some authorities, there is ample support for Freud's contention that orgasm in a psychologically mature woman is centered in the vagina, while in the adolescent girl (or emotionally immature woman) orgasm is achieved primarily through stimulation of the clitoris. Freud theorized that with the attainment of womanhood the center of orgasm moves to the vagina. However, since there is no way to "prove" such a hypothesis, and no physiological evidence to support the idea of a vaginal orgasm, the more biologically oriented sexologists have rejected it. Nevertheless, many psychologists and psychoanalysts who have studied sexuality from the approach of depth psychology, are convinced that there are, in fact, two types of orgasm, and that they are qualitatively, and not merely quantitatively, distinct. Perhaps the argument could be resolved if we had words to describe these very different experiences other than calling them "clitoral" and "vaginal," since these descriptions imply that it is merely a matter of the anatomical locus of sensation and that somehow this is what is important. It isn't. For that matter, to stress the importance of any sort of orgasm for its own sake makes little sense. The occurrence of vaginal orgasm is only important if it indicates something about her and her marriage. Unless we keep it in this perspective, it may become emphasized for its own sake. And this, in turn, may lead to a further development of the "sexual mystique" so prevalent in the writings of contemporary novelists.

For our purposes, we suggest the word "complete"

rather than "vaginal." Or perhaps the word *total* would be more descriptive of the mature female orgasm. It is an orgasm which starts deep within her body—subjectively, at least, in the vagina—and extends, as it increases in intensity, to every part of her body, seemingly to the tips of her fingernails. At its peak, her whole being seems to dissolve and she experiences an indescribable feeling of fulfillment and transcendence. She feels a loss of her ego boundaries as her entire being flows into him. It is an experience of such profoundness and meaning that no analogy is adequate to describe it, an experience which pervades and affects every aspect of her relationship with her husband, and one which makes the male orgasm seem almost rudimentary by comparison.

Sad to say, we believe only a minority of wives achieve this type of orgasm. If so, this is unfortunate since it indicates that too few marriages have grown in the way in which they should. Why, one might ask, should such an inference be drawn from an experience which plays such a small part in the total relationship of marriage? The answer rests in the psychology of woman. We often see women who, having read of such an orgasm, seek professional help in achieving it. One of the first things we explain, however, is that achievement of orgasm can never, in and of itself, be their goal. Recently, one such wife told us she wanted to learn how to experience total orgasm because she felt it would help what she described as her "mediocre" marriage. From the history she gave, it had probably been far worse than mediocre; a marriage marked by rivalry and bitterness almost from the beginning. During the initial visit, we explained to her the significance of the orgasm and the mistake she was making in confusing "cause" and "effect." The experience is not one which aids in the achievement of a good marriage; it *results* from a good marriage! It can never be approached directly since this would be antithetical to the nature of woman. It can be achieved *only* if the wife is able to *totally give herself* to her husband.

We don't feel the magnitude of this surrender of self can be exaggerated. We haven't heard a more dramatic— or accurate—description than the following, given by a truly "fulfilled" wife: "A woman must have complete faith and trust in her husband in order for it to happen. It's somewhat as if you were flying in an airplane with him and he asked that you step out to get him a cup of coffee and you did so without hesitation; this is the amount of trust that's necessary." Is it any wonder, then, that few wives have experienced it? How many feel this secure?

As we write this, we can hear the chorus of women asking how many husbands merit this degree of faith. And all we can answer is, probably none. No human being, male or female, could possibly do anything to *warrant* such complete trust. It simply cannot be *earned*. But it can be *given*. A wife is able to place this complete trust in her husband not because of what he is, but because of what she has become: *a woman*.

First, she must feel a deep sense of security, a sureness of self, and a satisfaction in her womanhood. In order to totally surrender, she must feel secure enough to overcome some very natural apprehensions. Her husband may increase her security, but it must originate with her. We have said that in order for a wife to love as a woman, she must step off a cliff, and it is with confidence that her husband will be there to catch her that she does so. No woman can give herself to this extent, however, if she fears that she will be "destroyed" or "swallowed up" if she does, and, unfortunately, this is a fairly apt description of the feelings of some wives. They fear they will lose their identity, and this is no trivial fear. Therefore, as they approach the brink of total orgasm, they near-panic, and they pull back and turn off the feelings. If a woman can't like herself and can't find joy in being a woman, she will be frozen by a fear that stems from her feelings of vulnerability, and shows itself in an inability to "let go." In Chapter XII we will return to the problem of frigidity and its causes. At this point, however, it might be well to clarify what is meant by frigidity. By way of definition, we must conclude that a wife is frigid unless she regularly achieves vaginal, or "total," orgasm in sexual relations with her husband, even though she may reach clitoral orgasm. We recognize this as a far more stringent definition than that employed by many writers, but it is the only definition that places sexuality within the content of the whole marriage and in keeping with the nature of a woman. We also recognize that by this definition, the majority of wives are frigid!

Much more than a man, a woman's sexual satisfaction is tied to her self-image. Also, her sexual fulfillment pervades her total existence to a greater extent. Her satisfaction doesn't terminate with the love-making; it continues into the following day or days as a sort of afterglow which eases the pressures of her many responsibilities and adds to the *joie de vivre* which is so much a part of womanhood. Thus, the observation that a woman, after making love, awakens with a song.

There are many emotional needs served by marital relations; tension reduction is only one, but an important one. The structure of our daily lives is such that few of us can escape the pressure and tension which comes from many sources, job, home, parenthood, neighbors, finances, etc. If the pressures are great and the individual has not developed adequate means of coping with them, the escape employed may be maladaptive and may lead only to problems which then create further pressures. Perhaps the most obvious example is excessive drinking, but there are many more which may be less apparent. Sexual pursuits may become a maladaptive attempt to escape just as much as alcohol. It may be used to meet neurotic as well as healthy needs, but here we are concerned only with the normal emotional needs and desires of husband and wife which are met in the marital union. In a good marriage, one in which both have found meaning and a mature sense of reality, the couple find a refuge—even though temporary—from the cares and anxieties which accompany life. It isn't accurate to call this an "escape." Nor a tranquilizer. It is part of the gift which they receive in return for their giving. It is part of the wonderful mystery of sexual love. We have always called it our "green valley." It may serve as a "weekend away from housework," or even a "vacation on a tropic isle," but, whatever, it provides an emotional peace and gives a renewed vigor to meet the challenge we each face. We feel it is important that this be said. We are all surrounded, at times nearly smothered, by responsibilities which too often have a way of becoming pressures. We cannot escape these responsibilities, and we wouldn't wish to do so. But we may be able to escape the pressure. And we should. And what more lovely way to escape to a green valley than together through our love-making.

It should go without saying that sexual relations should never be merely "used" to reduce anxiety, although we sometimes see couples who are guilty of this. Their marriage is nothing more than a neurotic interaction; it bears little relationship to love. To recognize and appreciate the fact that love-making is tension reducing in a good marriage, however, is not neurotic. It is one of the many gifts of marital sexuality. Our love-making at all times reflects our total life experience and the changing emotional climate of our life together. We may at one time turn to each other in joy; another time we may seek consolation in sorrow, reassurance in fear, or sympathy in disappointment.

No one could possibly analyze all the various emotional needs which are met in the sexual union. What becomes most apparent as a couple achieve success in their marriage is the unifying effect of the marital embrace. It acts as a "catalyst," dissolving the minor differences and irritations which might otherwise pull them apart. Being what we are as human beings, living in somewhat unique psychological worlds, there will be irritations and disagreements which may widen the gap which always exists between man and wife. But in loving each other, we can't tolerate being apart for long and we look for ways to close this painful distance. What could be more natural at such a time than the reuniting which is symbolized in lovemaking? We are not saying that arguments are settled through sexual relations, but rather that the separation which results from a disagreement—the feeling of apartness which lingers even after the differences have been settled —will very naturally draw the couple together sexually in an effort to again find the oneness they temporarily lost. To make love while still holding feelings of bitterness and hostility, however, is a contradiction in terms, and yet sadly enough we see couples who interrupt their fighting only long enough to have sexual relations, and then resume the battle. This seems to us more a perversion than an act of love! It makes the act a lie and an offense against all that is beautiful and holy in marriage. How then does it differ from a perversion?

To say that sexual love touches all dimensions of the marriage, that it colors the total relationship of husband and wife, and that it meets innumerable conscious and unconscious needs, is to state what should be obvious. Only human beings are capable of sexual love; and only human beings are capable of profaning sexual love. To describe this love solely in terms of pleasure or to think of it only as a "relief of concupiscence," is to profane a love which, like all love, mirrors the Divine.

The psychology of sexual love is the psychology of man and woman. All that we have been, all that we are, and all that we hope to become, will affect this love and be reflected in it. And if it is loving, we will find in it something above and beyond its mere humanness, but without ever rejecting the wonderful humanity of it.

CHAPTER X

Love-making: The Spiritual Experience

EACH OF THE sacraments can be called a "sacrament of love." Baptism, in which we are accepted into the loving arms of His church; Penance, with its promise of His never-ending mercy; Holy Eucharist, in which He gives the totality of His love to us, all are gifts of love. And God *is* love. In the sacrament of Matrimony, husband and wife are called to share in His love through a very wonderful and mysterious vocation. They are called *by* God to a union *in* God.

Just as in the other sacraments, in Christian marriage there is a continuing outward sign of an infusion of grace. It is the conjugal love expressed in the sexual union. This act is a symbol of the triune relationship of husband, wife, and God, one which mirrors the triune love of Father, Son and Holy Spirit. But how do we experience this? We may be told that the marital union is a source of grace, but how do we feel it, how do we discover His presence in this union?

As children we learn that God gives us grace and we have only to accept it. Or we may hear of God "filling" us with grace. Many of us grow up with a vague notion of grace as a mysterious "something" poured into us like water filling a pitcher. Perhaps this is why many say they have never experienced the *feeling* of God's grace. They simply don't know what to expect.

We aren't theologians, and any discourse on the nature of grace is beyond our knowledge and capabilities. We will leave it to them to define and distinguish *actual, sanctifying,* and *sacramental* grace. We feel certain, however, that none of the theologians or Christian philosophers hold that grace is an invisible substance of a sort which is injected into our souls. We prefer to think of it as the presence of God. And the experience of grace is the experience of God's presence with, for, and in us. It isn't some "thing" which He gives us; it is His gift of Himself.

When husband and wife repeat the words which mutually administer the sacrament of Matrimony, they can feel very confident. They have the promise of God that He will give them all the help they will need in order to achieve a fulfilled Christian marriage. He gives them a blank check. All they need do is be open to receive Him, to listen for the answers He will give to the question of how to best love. The answer will always come; we only fail to hear it when our own voice becomes so loud that our ears are deafened to His voice.

In sexual love, God very clearly reveals Himself. But perhaps in no other human activity is He less visible for many. How many wives (or husbands), if they were asked to recall the moment in the week when they felt closest to Christ, would answer, "When we made love"? In discussing the *spiritual* experience of sexual love, we often run into incredulity and occasionally, even hostility. (One highly indignant matron accused us of heresy and sacrilege!) Typical were the views of a very "pious" couple married nine years. They both admitted that the marital union is holy (they had heard it said a number of times), but they had never found any personal spiritual experience in the act. As the wife expressed it, "I could never feel the spiritual feeling during intercourse that I feel in church." Her husband felt the same, unfortunately. Since marriage is their sole vocation, however, and it is, to be sure, a religious vocation, how can they expect to find Christ anywhere unless they can find Him in their vocation? It seems to us that unless they can find Christ in their marital love, they stand little chance of finding Him in a church.

When we speak of finding Christ in the marital union, we are talking about a personal encounter. It is an emotional experience of a spiritual nature which accompanies the love-making in a mature marriage. This is, of course, highly subjective. So in attempting to describe it, we can only talk of what we have found it to be, and what others have told us it has meant to them. This is psychological, not theological; it isn't describing God, but our experience in trying to know Him through our marriage.

In Christian marriage, it seems Christ has given us a very natural bridge toward finding Him, "natural" in the sense that it is so in keeping with the nature of man and woman. The bridge, of course, is the one to whom we are joined; we each find our way to Christ through the other. Of course, married or unmarried, we can only experience Christ, and show love for God, if we are able to love persons. In marriage, the primary direction of our love should at all times be clear. The often conflicting obligations toward others which those in the single state may face, should be much less vexing to the married. All obligations to others must be viewed within the context of the marriage, and in relation to the primary obligation owed to one's spouse. This is the way in which we build the bridge. We strengthen it as we increase our marital unity. The more we are *present* for each other, the more He is *present* to us. We can't feel that this is just one way in which a husband or wife find Christ; we believe it is the *only* way.

If He doesn't become more real to us through our vocation, where else can we look?

We have several times spoken of the marital union as a renewal of the marriage vows. This is what a couple *should* experience, but many don't. Admittedly, it is an ideal, but an ideal is the only goal worth striving for. The fact that we may never attain our ideal, does not invalidate the ideal. In fact, an ideal, we might say, is by definition unattainable. For this very reason, it motivates us to continue striving toward it. If we settle for anything short of it, we stand still—and we atrophy. We had an ideal when we entered marriage. Hopefully, we haven't discarded it.

In the sealing of the marriage bond, we each promised to "take" the other, to "have and to hold, from this day forward, for better, for worse, for richer, for poorer, in sickness and in health, until death do us part." We pledged a *total* commitment, and it is this commitment which is symbolized physically in the marital act. This pledge is extensive, and the entire marriage rests upon its implications. It might be well, therefore, to consider what it means.

As a point of departure, let's look at the issue of sexual relations outside of marriage. There has been a great deal of discussion recently of the so-called "new morality." Its proponents claim that the moral values of our society are outmoded and unrealistic. Some even contend that the "traditional" moral values are detrimental to emotional health (a view shared by very few psychotherapists). Questions on these issues are now being publicly debated by high school as well as college groups. Although it may be worded in many different ways, the question most often raised paraphrases one of the principal arguments of these self-styled modern moralists: "Since the sexual act is an act of love, why, if the couple love each other and are mature enough to make such a decision, should it be considered morally wrong before marriage?"

Several answers might be offered. For one, we might seriously question the assumption that pre-marital sexual intercourse can ever be an act of love. Since the love is to desire that which is *good* for the other, an act which is immoral could not possibly be loving. But this answer would be begging the question, since the issue is whether, in fact, the act is immoral. We may still, nevertheless, raise the issue of loving. We have found, in discussing the issue, that most of the proponents of this view implicitly define love as little more than a positive attraction toward someone of the opposite sex. In other words, they see love as an *emotion*, nothing else. To them, love is not the gift of self, only the experience of certain positive feelings. And so, by their definition, it could be an act of love. If, on the other hand, love is seen as giving—and, hence, as a reflection of the perfection of giving, God's love for man—the assumption that the sexual union prior to marriage is an act of love is invalid. One or both are seeking solely to satisfy their own desires, regardless of what feeling they may have for each other. This makes the act exploitive; and exploitation is the antithesis of loving. Even though the desire may be shared and they may attempt to give sexual pleasure to each other, the act is still exploitive.

It is exploitive because in the act there is an implied promise and, prior to marriage or outside of marriage, this commitment cannot be made. The sexual act communicates not only the gift of self to the other but also the promise that this gift is irrevocable, that it is a gift of self *for a lifetime*. When we recite our vows, we are publicly acknowledging this promise. Outside of marriage, this can be nothing but a false promise.

The marital union is an act of love, but it has a very special character, one which distinguishes it from all other acts of love: It is a procreative act. Implied in the act is the promise of conception, and the pledge to each other to assume all of the responsibilities this entails. In receiving the gift of his wife's body, the husband gives his promise to cherish and protect, with his life if necessary, her and the child which may be the fruit of their union. She, likewise, implies an acceptance of the responsibilities of parenthood, and an acceptance of the child he gives her. This need not be (and probably often is not) a consciously recognized acceptance. Consciously or unconsciously, however, this acceptance of responsibility, the pledge of their lives to each other and to the children which may be born of their love, is implied in their sexual union. In thus giving to each other in love, they renew again and again the vows of the vocation to which they were called and to which they give witness. Needless to say, experiencing the sexual union as a renewal of vows does not result from merely being told that this is what the act *should* symbolize and this is what husband and wife *should* experience. Even with a loving marriage and healthy attitudes, they may not perceive it as a mutual pledge of fidelity, since experiencing it as a renewal of vows will not stem from a conscious decision to do so but, rather, it will result from the maturing of the marriage. That is, it is a *product* of loving, not an act of will. Don't ask us how this occurs. We only know that it does. It's another of the wonderful, unexplainable, rewards.

Many couples who have found joy and fulfillment in Christian marriage have spoken of the orgasm as a moving spiritual experience. This should hardly be surprising since it is at this moment that husband and wife are most completely "joined in one flesh." Little wonder that such a profound sensual experience of mutual orgasm may take on a mystical character. Certainly, its description in terms of an experience of transcending spirituality, as "a glimpse of the Beatific Vision," sounds the rhapsodic tones of mysticism. As one wife described it: "At the moment of climax, when I feel my husband flow into me, it's like a tremendous infusion of grace."

Such an admission might raise more than a few eyebrows in either disbelief or shock. After all, there are still writings in print which warn of the danger of "spiritualizing" sexuality. It should be kept in mind, however, that what we are discussing is not a theology of sexuality, but rather the spiritual experience which accompanies sexual love. To speak of this spiritual experience is not to deify the act. And to say that we find God's presence in lovemaking is not to assert that the sexual union *is* God! In a similar manner, we might very well talk of feeling God's presence in the beauty of a forest without embracing pantheism.

Spirituality, like sexuality, can never rightfully be considered merely a part of the marriage, distinct from all other parts. We simply cannot compartmentalize spirituality, or, for that matter, any other aspect of our life. And yet many couples seek to find God apart from their relationship to each other just as they separate devotion to Him from their work, recreation, and sexual love. We have talked with scores of couples for whom this is true, couples who have never knelt together in prayer, who have never held hands during mass, who have never sought spiritual guidance *as a couple*.

They miss two important points: first, that the very essence of marriage makes the prayer of husband or wife a mutual prayer, and second, that mutual prayer, freely expressed in their own words, provides a meaningful channel of communication between them and a deepening of their union in God.

Prayer is the directing of one's thoughts and actions toward God; it is a striving to relate to God, to increase His *presence.* If we think of conjugal prayer in these terms, we should have little difficulty recognizing the marital union as a profound prayer. In turning to each other in sexual love, the couple turn toward God. Their act of love becomes a profession of faith, and of hope, as they give themselves in cooperation with His plan. No human activity gives more glory to man's creator than the act by which man is permitted to share in creation. As the marriage bond deepens, the couple become increasingly aware of this. Their life together, their "works, joys, and sufferings," takes on the beauty and the mystery of prayer. In a marriage which has matured in love and become centered in Christ, the day-by-day cycle of activity is not only offered as prayer, it is experienced as prayer. They need not be told that the marital union is "a most loving prayer." They *live* it.

Living the vocation of conjugal love brings all other sacraments into focus. Many couples have spoken of the differences in the way in which they approach the sacraments of Penance and Holy Eucharist that have come with the growth of their marriages. They no longer go into the confessional seeking merely absolution; they look for spiritual direction in loving their spouses, and Christ's presence in the sacrament to aid them in loving. They have learned that virtue is not a mere absence of vice, that Christianity—and their Christian marriage—is a call to perfection, and it is aid in striving toward this perfection that they seek in the sacrament of Penance. It is the obligations of marriage which are carried into the confessional, the failure to love which is confessed, the grace to love more which is sought.

The reception of Christ's body in the Holy Eucharist is a social act. It unites us with Christ in the loving sacrifice of His redemptive act, and it unites us one to another. In the sacrament of Baptism, we become a part of Christ's

Mystical Body, joined in union with all Christians under the headship of Christ. When we, as members of His Mystical Body, brothers and sisters in Christ, receive Him in the Holy Eucharist, our bond becomes even more evident to us; it is an act of *communion*—an "act of sharing." In and through the Body of Christ we become *one*. In sexual love, husband and wife become *one*. Here, also, it is Christ, the catalyst, fusing the separate identities into a single body. As our marriage grows in Christ-centeredness, the unity which we feel as we kneel together to receive the Blessed Sacrament and the unity which we experience in marital relations both increase, the one reinforcing the other, and together they become a single experience of oneness.

Recognizing, on an intellectual level, the holiness of the marital union, and *experiencing* spirituality in the conjugal act are not the same thing. Most Christian couples, we feel sure, would agree that marital relations are blessed by God, but few can say they experience a benediction in the act. Why? Probably, two reasons: First of all, marital sexuality is seldom presented as a spiritual encounter. As children, we learned only a negative view. Parents, in their concern with the dangers of sexual immorality, stressed *sin*, and little else. The marital union has not sufficiently been presented as an act of virtue and a means of giving glory to God. But there is another, more important, reason. Discovering the presence of Christ in the sexual union is a reward which is found not in a blinding flash of insight, but through gradual awareness, paralleling the growth of husband and wife toward the goal of mutual sanctity. It is the marriage, the total relationship, which must mature. There is always the danger that breaking the marriage up, even for purposes of discussion, into "physical," "psychological," and "spiritual" aspects may lead us into the error of seeing man as merely a composite of roles, interests, or personality dimensions, and life and marriage in the same way, a point we have made several times, but one we feel needs restatement. The *whole* marriage grows, or no growth takes place. Husband and wife come to *know* Christ, to *love* Him, and to *see* Him in their sexual union, as they strive to *know love*, and *see* each other. Finding Christ in the marriage, like finding happiness, is not an objective which can be approached directly. Both *result* from loving. This is a truth which should be almost immediately apparent, especially to a Christian couple, but experience has shown us that it is not. Instead, many have accepted happiness as the goal of life—and of marriage—and have become obsessed with "searching" for happiness. Usually, they confuse pleasure with happiness, and in doing so, never manage to find happiness, God, or any fulfillment in their marriage. As they fill their lives with distractions, they fail to discover the mystery and paradox of love: only as we give fully of ourselves to another, does God become present in our lives, and only then do we find happiness.

We feel very inadequate, very humble, and somewhat uneasy in writing of the spiritual experience in sexual love since it is so subjective, so personal an experience, and we have had so few sources upon which to draw other than our own introspections. While we have talked at length with other couples of what they have found, so few have admitted to *any* spiritual experience in their sexual union, we are reluctant to generalize. This, then, has been our experience, the only experience we can speak for with validity. Whatever others may have experienced, however, we feel confident that He will reveal Himself in this union. We have only to open our eyes and ears to each other—and to Him.

CHAPTER XI

Pregnancy and Sexual Love

"PREGNANCY IS a nine-month extension of the orgasm," was the way one happily married wife described it. No poet could say it better; no philosopher could find in it more profound meaning. It is exactly that, an extension of the sexual love to its ultimate fruition.

And yet today, even among Christian couples, there is a tendency to view sexual love and procreation as distinct, and to assert the primacy of mutual love apart from, and even to the exclusion of, procreation. The sexual union, they say, is an act of love, and it need not be associated with procreation. They reject what they consider a purely biologistic concept of sexuality, and many reject procreation as one of the ends of marriage.

Even many moral theologians, until recently, fell into a similar type of dichotomous thinking. They also made a distinction between love and procreation in seeking to understand the place of Christian sexuality. "The procreation and education of children" was held to be the primary end of marriage; the couple's spiritual and emotional growth in love was relegated, at least by implication, to a secondary (and less important) position.

Both extremes, however, convey the same mistaken impression: that sexual love, as an act of love, and sexual love, as an act of procreation, can be separated. And in either case, the necessary conclusions which follow such compartmentalized thinking rob the marital union of its highest dignity.

If we are to find fulfillment in marital love and discover its proper place in the redeemed state, we must reject any suggestion that the two can be separate, since the one extreme, in approaching sexuality hedonistically, denies the sanctity given it by God, and the other extreme, stressing a biologistic cause and effect, detracts from the dignity of human love. There can never rightfully be an argument of "primary" and "secondary"—the two are one and inseparable. *Conception, and the procreation of a child, is the fulfillment of sexual love; it is the implied promise of the marital union, the ordained fruition of the marital bond.* Just as the sperm and ovum fuse and develop in the miracle of conception, the seeds of love fuse, grow, and blossom during the nine months in which, together, husband and wife co-operate in God's plan to bring their child to the maturity of birth. As the marriage deepens in love, His plan seems to unfold and become clear. Arguments about primary and secondary ends then seem meaningless. For such a husband and wife, the marital union is clearly an act of *procreative love.*

Does this then mean that the couple come together in the sexual embrace only when they desire to conceive a child? Yes and no. We are *not* saying that a couple should or must consciously desire another child in order for the act to be licit. Nor are we in any way suggesting that the marital union is licit only if conception is possible, nor even that it is most meaningful or fulfilling only at these times. Definitely not! But rather, we are re-emphasizing what has been said before: as the love between husband and wife deepens, they each become increasingly aware of the need they feel to share in the conception of a child.

It is a need to impregnate and to be impregnated which is rooted in the core of their natures as man and woman and which manifests itself through loving and the desire to become *one*. It is, in fact, this desire for oneness which makes the sexual union and procreation psychologically so inseparable. It is *him* she is carrying in her womb as she carries his child and in this way, the union which is formed as they come together in coitus continues, without the emptiness and the pain of separation as they part. The oneness which is climaxed in their mutual orgasm takes tangible form in the new life—a part of each of them— which grows within her body. It is their love which develops within her; and it is their love which is witnessed in the birth of their child.

There may, of course, be financial or physical reasons which would make another pregnancy undesirable and perhaps even feared, but this does not in any way contradict what we have said. Even where circumstances would make another pregnancy inadvisable, there is an unconscious—or perhaps even conscious—desire for impregnation on the part of both husband and wife. They may deny or suppress such emotional needs, but in doing so they stand to lose something very precious. Moreover, they both lose, and in more than a single way. It might be well for us to look at some of these ways and the effects they have on the marriage.

The wife may deny her emotional need to be impregnated; she may even view childbearing as a cross imposed by the more fortunate male and by God (also a male, no doubt). But the sexual act will then usually be far less than fulfilling for her since she perceives it as an act of masculine exploitation. This can only result in a loss of the total enjoyment which should be found in the marital union. There is something more, however. She also stands to lose her love for her husband and his love for her be her hostility and resentment, regardless of how much she may attempt to hide it. By rejecting his child, she rejects him. She may, of course, deny this and claim that it is not her husband that she is rejecting, only an undesired pregnancy, but in denying her need for his child, she is denying her need for him. What she says, in effect, is, "I will not conceive a child *with* you; you will have to force a child *on* me, and I will then reject you as the father and the child will be mine alone." Should she become pregnant, she will manifest her resentment in making sure that the pregnancy is a nine-month ordeal for her husband as well as herself. Seldom will she permit a day to go by without reminding him of the suffering he has inflicted upon her. And, since our physical reactions are so closely tied to our emotional states, she probably will, in fact, experience a "difficult" pregnancy and a "difficult" delivery. Psychoanalysts, for example, have long pointed out the relationship between severe problems of vomiting in pregnancy and the unconscious desire to rid oneself of the unwanted fetus. Regardless, however, of how real or fictitious her suffering, one can be sure that she will whine and complain throughout the pregnancy, never permitting it to become a period of joy for her and her husband and a period of growth for their marriage.

If such a wife were to admit her need to be impregnated, she would have to give up one of the more potent weapons she employs against her husband, the accusation that the pregnancy, with the discomfort that accompanies it, is all "his fault." She could no longer take satisfaction in resenting what she herself desired, and she might then be forced toward the insight that it is not her husband or the masculine role that she resents, but her own sex. This is, understandably, not easy to accept; it is far more comfortable to direct her hostility outward—toward him—than inward—toward herself. In doing so, however, she loses, in the long run, the opportunity to become fully a woman.

Should the husband, rather than the wife, reject or deny the need to impregnate, the effect on the marriage will be at least as harmful. In submission to him, the wife communicates her acceptance of *his* child. This is her gift, the gift of her life to him and to his child. What greater gift could she give? If, then, he denies the desire to reciprocate with his gift, the need to have her carry and give birth to their child, and the acceptance of the responsibility of fatherhood, he is repudiating her love, her "gift of self."

This may not be a conscious, or even intended, rejection. But it is, nevertheless, a rejection of her. It makes the act of love convey a contradictory message: "I love you; but I don't *love* you."

He may be expressing his fears and insecurity. The responsibility that is assumed in the conception and birth of a child is formidable, and it may be frightening to the husband who lacks courage and self-confidence. The fear of responsibility may cause him to suppress his need for procreation just as a woman's fear of the discomfort of pregnancy and pain of childbirth may rob her of the joy of anticipation and acceptance of conception.

The fear of pregnancy can, of course, be very real—and very severe. Complications in prior pregnancies, serious financial problems, even the terror instilled by the tales of old wives, may create serious difficulties which impede marital growth, difficulties which have no simple solution overcoming any deep fear is a challenging task. Where the fear is rooted in other than just present reality problems such as physical or financial difficulties (and sometimes even then), professional counseling may be advised. Where, however, the fear stems from egocentricity and an unwillingness to give oneself, husband and wife might do well to keep in mind the words of the apostle John, "Love casts out fear."

Sexual relations seldom cease during pregnancy. Most couples continue to have intercourse throughout pregnancy and, barring certain physical complications which might make it inadvisable, most physicians find nothing harmful in this (although most medical authorities advise against it during the last weeks). Problems other than physical may arise, however. Some wives report a loss of sexual desire during this period, especially during the first three or four months. Infrequently, this approaches a strong aversion to all sexual contact. These women become, at least for a time, totally frigid.

Biochemical or hormonal changes which accompany pregnancy may partly account for these changes, but fear or resentment of the pregnancy usually has much to do with this loss of erotic response. Should the wife blame her husband for what she feels she is being forced to undergo, she may be unable to give herself to him in the fullness necessary to achieve sexual satisfaction. Thus, the first step if a wife finds herself "temporarily frigid" during pregnancy should be a self-examination, a thorough probing of her reactions and feelings toward the pregnancy, her husband, and her own sexuality.

Fatigue which accompanies pregnancy may also play a major part in diminishing sexual response. Many, although not all, women experience extreme fatigue, especially during the first and last trimesters of pregnancy. Hence, although a mother-to-be may feel no lessening of sexual desire, the end of the day may find her too tired to adequately respond in love-making. If both husband and wife understand it, and attempt, through loving, to adjust to it and, at least to the extent possible, relieve the fatigue, it need not become a problem. Even more than usual, the husband can "take over" many of the wife's chores, giving

her more help with the housework and children, carrying
her over the rough spots that drain her of energy. For her
part, she may attempt to pace herself, to be as rested as
possible for the moments they have together.

As she grows and increases in size, the wife may find
that some positions for intercourse are uncomfortable. Pressure on the abdomen or deep penetration of the vagina
may also make some positions inadvisable during the latter months of pregnancy. Ordinarily, however, the couple
will have little difficulty discovering positions that will be
comfortable and which will permit a full expression of
their sexual love.

In this, as in so much else during the pregnancy, the
husband bears a major responsibility. Seldom in marriage
is more tenderness and loving consideration demanded of
him. In recognizing and accepting his role during pregnancy, he accepts the paternity of his child and witnesses
the highest form of conjugal love. The almost impossible
burden that so many wives find in childbearing would be
lifted and pregnancy would become for them a period
of joy and formation in love if their husbands viewed the
pregnancy as a shared experience. In God's plan for Christian marriage, the child is conceived and born in love
and it is in love that *both* husband and wife, not the wife
alone, carry the child and together bring it into the world.

The husband fills more than the role of helpmate to his
wife during pregnancy. He provides the reassurance and
emotional support necessary to carry her through the nine
months with flying colors. He understands the feeling of
vulnerability she experiences during pregnancy, the need
she has, even more than before, to know that she is safe,
protected by the love with which he surrounds her. Many
women have been "prepared" for pregnancy by other
wives, embittered women who talked of husbands who
supposedly lost interest in their wives when a child was

expected. Young brides, filled with joyful anticipation are taught that a woman's body in pregnancy is sexually unattractive, even ugly, that they can no longer "hold" their husbands by physical charms. The fears that result may be hard to extinguish, especially so if they are reinforced by a callous or inattentive husband. In a marriage of love, however, the husband finds his wife no less attractive when she is carrying his child. Instead, he watches her take on a new, often mysterious, beauty and a dimension of sexuality which marks her fulfillment as a woman. And in a thousand ways, large and small, he communicates this to her.

With each succeeding month of the pregnancy, the child growing within its mother becomes more *real,* more a *person,* to its parents. This is a period which offers an opportunity for great growth in the marriage. The changes which signal the development of their child, the first fluttering movements of life, the hard kicks of a healthy infant, the first contractions of labor, draw the couple ever closer together. The patience and understanding of both should grow with the pregnancy and add increments to their union, building blocks of love and communication. The hours spent in planning and dreaming for their child are incomparable hours of oneness.

The onset of labor brings a new, and awesome closeness to their sexual love. With the birth of each child, the relationship of husband and wife changes; it never remains the same. Whether or not the period of labor and delivery serves to deepen their bond, however, will depend upon the closeness they attained during the pregnancy. Hopefully, they will share an experience of unity in the birth of their child as they did in the sexual love in which it was conceived. Perhaps at no time in their life together is it more important that they be together. We have listened to wives bitterly recall years later having been left alone during their hours of labor. Often it was the doctor who suggested to the husband that he "go home and get some rest"; at times, the wife has been the one to urge her husband to leave. In any case, she remembers only that he was not by her side when she needed him, and the beauty and joy that could have been theirs had he stood beside her is forever lost. An increasing number of obstetricians and hospitals are recognizing the benefit of husband and wife sharing in the birth, and are therefore permitting, and even encouraging, the husband to be present during the delivery. Even where it is not possible for him to be present in the delivery room, however, the husband will want to be as close as possible to his wife, both physically and emotionally, throughout the labor and delivery; if he is not permitted in the delivery room, he will at least be by her side until the time of delivery, and be waiting to greet her and their child.

With the birth of each child, the cycle of human life is renewed, and the adventure and responsibility of parenthood is begun again. Each time it is a unique experience. Regardless of whether it be the first child or the sixth, its introduction into the family changes the structure of the family and all the complex interactions of the members. Thus, each successive child makes his or her distinct contribution to the other members of what St. John Chrysostom called the "Church in Miniature."

The newborn infant offers an opportunity to understand something of love and the emotions which accompany love. Very often we have listened to someone ask, "How can I give myself to him (or her) if I don't *feel* any love?" The question, however, reveals a basic error. Love is *not* a feeling or an emotion; it is a volitional act, an act of will whereby we give of ourselves. To be sure, when we say "I love you" we are expressing an emotion, but the emotion accompanies the loving; it is not, itself, love. The more we give of ourselves to another, the more positive emotions toward the person will grow, not from anything we receive *from* them, but from what we give *to* them. How often do we hear a husband or wife attempt to justify a lack of loving by the accusation: "How can I be expected to love her when she doesn't show any love for me?" And yet they will profess to love an infant who can give *nothing* in return. The loving emotion which a mother feels toward her baby is so accepted in our culture that many consider it to be an innate component of the feminine nature, so-called "mother love." Yet there is nothing innate in "mother love"; it stems from the total dependency of the child. The mother must meet all of the child's needs if the child is to survive, and in giving herself to the child, without asking or expecting anything in return, she experiences these profound feelings of warmth and tenderness toward her infant which we call "mother love." If husband and wife come to understand this love of parent for child, to see it as embodying the essence of human love, and its accompanying emotion, they may receive new and deeper insights into the conjugal love which gave their child life. And hopefully, they may discover a very important truth, one which goes to the core of the responsibilities of parenthood: The love they give their child, and the love and security that the child experiences, will be never more—nor less—than a reflection of the love they give to each other.

CHAPTER XII

Problems in Sexual Love

THERE ARE SOMETIMES barriers which stand in the way of sexual love. Most of them we erect by refusing to love and stubbornly remaining within an egocentric world. Other barriers, however, can be even more formidable, and they may arise in spite of a desire to love. They are what we usually term "sexual problems."

These problems may stem from either physical or psychological causes, but in most cases the psychological and the somatic interact so thoroughly that we speak of them as *psychosexual* problems. For our purposes, we choose to define these problems as any conditions, regardless of cause, which inhibit full sexual satisfaction or which impede the successful completion of the marital act. Either spouse may experience the problem, but in any case, it will affect both of them and their marriage. Most of these conditions can range from very mild to severe, and can be transitory, recurrent, or chronic.

It might be better to call some of these "problems in sexual adjustment," rather than "sexual problems." In the first months of marriage, many couples experience difficulties in marital relations which may have the same symptoms as some of the more serious conditions. This shouldn't cause concern, however. Usually time and experience will resolve these initial difficulties if they are not overemphasized and blown up into a real problem. Should the symptoms persist, the couple can then, but only then, be said to be suffering from a sexual problem. With this distinction in mind, let's briefly describe the more commonly encountered sexual difficulties.

IMPOTENCE

Impotence (or impotency), is the inability of an adult male to perform intercourse, that is, the inability to maintain an erection until successful completion of the marital act. It may occur under a variety of conditions. A husband, for example, may be potent at the beginning of intercourse and become impotent before the act is completed. Or, he may be fully aroused, with an erection, during preliminary love-making only to experience an impotency reaction at the initiation of coitus.

Impotence may be either organic or functional (i.e., psychological), but in any case, it is a symptom of a condition. And it is the condition which should be treated. Organically, it may result from injury to the central nervous system, either the brain or spinal cord, or from a number of various diseases including tuberculosis, leukemia, anemia, and diabetes. It may also be caused by hormonal abnormalities or by disorders of the genitourinary system. And, of course, nutritional deficiencies, fatigue, and the normal aging process will all affect the adequacy of sexual functioning. Where the cause is strictly physical, the impotency reaction can often be alleviated by medication, diet, or, in some cases, surgery. The first step, therefore, in the diagnosis and treatment of impotence should be a thorough physical examination.

In most cases, organic pathology will be ruled out by such an examination. *Psychological impotency* probably accounts for nine out of ten cases of male sexual inadequacy. But this doesn't mean that the husband with a psychological impotency reaction is necessarily suffering from a serious or deep-seated emotional disturbance. While such problems can result in impotency, occasional inability to maintain an erection and complete the sexual union may be due to a number of factors; and probably the majority of husbands have experienced occasional "failures."

If we recall the part played by the autonomic nervous system in male sexual arousal, we can rather easily understand the physiologic basis of impotency. To review briefly, the autonomic nervous system has two divisions: the *parasympathetic* system and the *sympathetic* system. In most cases, these "sub-systems" work antagonistically to one another; stimulation from the sympathetic system, for example, acts somewhat to "block" innervation from the parasympathetic system. Erection is a parasympathetic function. Thus, strong sympathetic stimulation during sexual arousal may obstruct the innervation necessary to sustain the erection. If we also recall that it is the sympathetic nervous system which is involved in the emotional reactions of fear, rage, or anxiety, we can easily understand how any stimulus which elicits such a reaction will also inhibit erection. Since the autonomic reaction is physiologically the same in both fear and rage, either may affect sexual adequacy; the emotion need not be directly related to sexuality itself.

For this reason, impotency can quickly grow from a single reaction into a major problem in which the man finds himself repeatedly incapable of sustaining an erection. This was clearly illustrated in the case of a salesman in his early forties. He returned from a trip, tense and exhausted after many hours of driving in heavy traffic. When his wife made sexual overtures, he felt obliged to respond.

Although they engaged in extensive preliminary love-making, he found he could achieve only a partial erection and consequently was unable to complete the act. His wife contributed to his feelings of chagrin and inadequacy by thoughtlessly expressing her frustration, thus adding to what became a problem. A day or two later he came across an article in one of the popular magazines for men which discussed the supposed decrease in sexual drive accompanying middle age. The article was exaggerated and misleading, but he had no way of knowing this. He, therefore, mistakenly concluded that his "failure" was due to aging. His anxiety was intense and that evening, when he attempted to "prove" his sexual adequacy by making love, he again couldn't keep an erection. The condition continued for several months before he sought professional help. Each time he attempted intercourse he became apprehensive; the fear of sexual failure would overwhelm him and, sure enough, he would find himself incapable of completing the act. Each time this occurred, it further increased his anxiety and, hence, increased the probability of its reoccurrence.

This causal chain of *impotence-fear-impotence* may begin on the honeymoon. With all the pressures and fatigue which so often accompany weddings, receptions, and honeymoon trips, many grooms find they are incapable of love-making on their wedding night. The inexperienced husband may also suffer from anxieties which add to the chances of "failure." In most cases, however, this is merely part of the adjustment process, and nothing to be concerned about. Time and experience will usually resolve the difficulty.

Where the impotency is more than a transitory happening, however, it can seriously impair the marriage. Since, in most cases, the problem can be alleviated, the husband has a serious obligation to take whatever steps are necessary to find a remedy. True psychological impotency may evidence any of a number of conscious or unconscious emotional difficulties. It is not within the scope of this book to go into the various psychodynamic factors which might produce the reaction. We can only advise that where such a problem appears to exist, the husband should seek some form of competent psychotherapeutic help. As in so many other areas of human suffering, there are an appalling number of quack cures, devices, and "rejuvenating" nostrums advertised to cure impotency. Where the problem is physical, however, only a physician is qualified to diagnose and treat it; where the cause is emotional, the patient should then be referred to a psychotherapist.

PREMATURE EJACULATION

An even more common difficulty, and one which often has similar psychological causes, is so-called *premature ejaculation.* In some men, ejaculation may take place before intromission; in others, it may occur almost immediately after entrance into the vagina. In either case, the problem is one of the husband achieving orgasm too quickly, that is, before the wife is ready and able to reach her climax. Since the question then is that of duration of coitus following intromission *in relation to the wife's orgasm,* one might start by asking, "How long *should* coitus continue after intromission?" It would be senseless, however, to attempt to answer such a question. It implies that some sort of norms exist that can be employed as criteria. Obviously, no such quantitative approach has any application. Kinsey and his associates found, with the group they interviewed, that the majority averaged two to five minutes between intromission and ejaculation. But this doesn't tell us anything that will aid any particular couple. Their goal should be mutual satisfaction in the completion of the marital union—satisfaction for them; and no statistical averages can help them achieve this end.

While some cases of premature ejaculation have been found to be related to physical causes, such as oversensitivity of the glans in some uncircumcised men, the vast majority are the result of various emotional factors. This does not mean that premature ejaculation is necessarily pathological. In most cases, it is not. Again we find that during the early months of marriage, overexcitement, anxiety, and inexperience often combine to make it extremely difficult, if not impossible, to retard orgasm.

Perhaps of greatest importance is the attitude of the wife. Should she respond with dramatic disappointment to his inability to retard ejaculation, she may rouse feelings of anxiety and self-reproach in him which will then act to increase the chances of a reoccurrence in much the same way we observe it in impotency reactions. Thus, any such reactions on her part may serve only to increase the likelihood of her own frustration in the future and will, of course, evidence a very real lack of loving. The husband, too, should view such an occurrence with calm good sense and rational attitudes. Inability to retard ejaculation is not a disaster; nor does it indicate a lack of manhood. Occasional premature ejaculation can become a problem, but only if husband and wife *make it a problem.*

Nevertheless, complete sexual satisfaction usually makes it desirable for both husband and wife to be able to retard (or at times accelerate) orgasm. This is frequently a matter of learning something of one's sexual responses and those actions which will retard or speed up the climax.

Perhaps the most effective means of reducing the chance of premature ejaculation is to increase the frequency of marital relations. This may seem a rather obvious point, but it is frequently overlooked by couples trying to attain mutual satisfaction in the tempo of their love-making. Initial intercourse following a lengthy period of abstinence will often be overly stimulating and will result in ejaculating too quickly. This experience is not at all uncommon, for example, the first time the couple have relations following the waiting period after the birth of a child (usually six weeks). As the couple then once again establish their usual frequency of intercourse, a mutually satisfying tempo of love-making is also re-established.

Like impotency reactions, premature ejaculations may occur on occasion without it indicating a problem, and if the couple have enjoyed a mutually fulfilling sexual relationship, they will not permit it to become a problem. But, also like impotency reactions, it can be emotionally traumatic to a husband if it occurs during the first days of marriage, masculine vanity being what it is. It may be particularly shattering if the groom has listened to the many "authorities" who built a mystique around the initial act of sexual intercourse, portraying it as *the* crucial experience in the marriage, one which will set the emotional tone of the entire relationship. It can, but only if the husband shows a total disregard for his wife. In many, perhaps most, cases, the first time the couple have sexual relations they may be less than fully successful, but sexual love is a growth process and a skill. The wedding night is only the beginning. The ability to retard ejaculation usually develops over a period of time, often a considerable period. If the problem continues, the husband should seek professional help, but if it is only a "problem of adjustment," some suggestions may be of benefit.

Many writers have suggested concentrating on other, presumably diverting, thoughts as a means of retarding ejaculation. One gave examples which included thinking about problems at work or mentally figuring out solutions to mathematical problems. Empirically, we know that this method can be shown to be effective in prolonging coitus. Climax is greatly dependent upon psychological stimulation, and it is a well-established psychological fact that, at any moment, we are able to fully concentrate on only a single thing. But it has seemed to us that such a technique, even though effective, is less than desirable. First of all, it suggests that the husband's sexual actions be deliberately very mechanical and impersonal, and that he self-sacrificingly forgo his enjoyment in order to give his wife satisfaction; second, that he emotionally removed himself from the sexual union. But this union implies a total involvement of husband and wife, and any preoccupation, whether intentional or unintentional, can only detract from the ultimate sexual fulfillment of both; not only the husband, but also the wife. Only the most self-centered woman would be unaffected by the knowledge that her husband was concentrating on mathematical equations while they made love!

If we view this advice in another way, however, it becomes not only an effective "technique" for prolonging ejaculation, but an essential approach to love-making. If, rather than concentrating on his own sexual feelings and reactions, the husband directs his thoughts and actions toward discovering the ways in which he can increase his wife's enjoyment, he may find it possible to retard orgasm and, at the same time, contribute to the growth of their sexual love. We might also call this a "distraction," but it is a distraction from egocentricity—and an egocentric love is not love.

Two further suggestions might be considered in attempting to learn how to prolong ejaculation. First, premature ejaculation, where the husband is able to effect intromission but ejaculates long before the wife reaches orgasm, is often due to inadequate pre-coital love-making. In Chapter VIII, we pointed out that it is the husband, ordinarily, who takes the initiative in the love-making; but it is the wife who has the responsibility of signaling when she is ready to complete the act. It is well to keep in mind that she alone is aware of her sexual arousal, its intensity, and how close she is to orgasm. If, then, the husband is striving to sexually *love* her, he will attempt to bring her close to the summit of orgasm before intromission, waiting for her to signal when she is ready to complete the act and achieve climax.

In addition, the couple should be aware that the wife may still reach orgasm even if the husband finds it impossible to continue coitus after ejaculation. Usually this can be achieved by stimulation of the clitoris without the penis having to be withdrawn from the vagina. Since the question sometimes is raised, the couple should be reassured that there is nothing morally wrong in this. It is morally permissible for the husband to stimulate the wife to climax either before or after his ejaculation.

Lastly, since the husband is usually the more active partner in the sexual act, an understanding of his movements in coitus is sometimes of help in overcoming premature ejaculation. Often, the husband can retard orgasm if he momentarily stops his movements when he feels that ejaculation is imminent. Intromission, the first thrust of the penis into the vagina, usually is intensely stimulating and, should the husband engage in deep thrusting movements at once, ejaculation may occur too soon. It is often of help, therefore, if the husband delays his movements immediately after entering until the excessive excitement partially subsides.

The kind of movements employed will also be important in accelerating and retarding ejaculation. Deep thrusting movements in which nearly the entire length of the penis moves in and out of the vagina provide maximal stimulation to the glans. Thus, if the husband wishes to prolong coitus, he might be wise to avoid these movements until both are ready for orgasm. Instead, lateral movements, in which the pelvis is moved from side to side while the penis remains fully inserted in the vagina, will usually not result in such extreme stimulation, yet will ordinarily give intense pleasure to the wife.

PROBLEMS OF FREQUENCY

Although it doesn't meet our definition of sexual problems, complaints over the frequency of marital relations are heard so often that some discussion seems called for. A spouse may express dissatisfaction that the other wants relations "too often" or "not often enough". And despite what some may think, the complaint of "not often enough" is heard as frequently from wives as from husbands.

Just as with so many other sexual disagreements, controversy over frequency of intercourse usually indicates more basic conflict in the marriage. This would seem obvious, and yet from time to time we come across an article which attributes such marital incompatibility to differences in physical make-up, the notion being that the sexual drive of one spouse greatly exceeds that of the other. This has almost no factual basis. The sexual drive, is, in part, directed by secretion of gonadotrophic hormones, but differences in the desired frequency of intercourse seldom are related to differences in such physiological factors (with the rare exception, of course, of a physical condition which severely impairs functioning of the endocrine system).

In attempting to work through such problems, we also enter a cul-de-sac if we ask, "How often *should* a couple have relations?" There can be only one answer to this question: as often as each desire to do so. If they are motivated to love, and make their marital act an act of love, the frequency of their desire for intercourse will determine what is "normal" for them. It may run anywhere from once a day to less than once each week. The important thing is whether they find the frequency of their sexual relations *mutually* satisfying—regardless of Kinsey's statistics.

If both hold healthy attitudes, and both are emotionally mature, any differences in desired frequency can be expected to iron out and a mutually satisfying "cycle" of marital relations established within the first few months of the marriage—assuming, again, that the couple seek *to love,* not merely *to be loved.*

In attempting to deal with the problem, it is often necessary to question further, in detail, the spouse voicing the complaint; the complaint "too often" or "too seldom" is ambiguous. We need to know what *this* husband or wife, subjectively, considers "too often" or "too seldom." And, since even a statement of frequency can be misleading, it is important to know something of the nature of their sexual relations. Recently, we spoke with a woman in her thirties, married fourteen years, who complained that her husband's sexual demands were totally unreasonable. "He wants intercourse at least once every day; sometimes twice, and this has always been true." A very different picture emerged, however, as we questioned her. "What you have told us is that your husband frequently expresses sexual desires, but how often do you actually have intercourse?" She admitted that she consented only about every week to ten days. Her husband sarcastically described their situation rather well: "I've learned that if I want relations once a week, I have to pester her for seven days." Later, in therapy, the wife related a bit of advice she had been given by her mother. "Once a week," mother had told her, "is all that should be required of any wife; a woman is a fool if she lets her husband take advantage of her more often than that." Carrying her mother's bitterness and hostility, she managed to avoid looking at herself and asking, "What is wrong with me?" It was much easier to shift the problem and the blame to her husband.

Where sexual demands are actually excessive, that is, where one of the spouses desires relations so often that the other is either physically fatigued or (in the case of the husband) finds it impossible to perform the act, we may be dealing with a neurotic symptom. Such a husband, for example, may be attempting to dispel unconscious fears of sexual inadequacy, or even be reacting to the anxiety of latent homosexuality. He may, in other words be trying to convince himself of his virility. Or a sexually demanding wife may be seeking constant reassurance of her husband's love in order to bolster her faltering self-image ("prove to me that you find me desirable and womanly"). In any case, one thing can be said with certainty: the individual, whether man or woman, who feels an excessive need for sexual relations is not achieving mature satisfaction in intercourse. A mutually fulfilling act of sexual love leaves both spouses with a satisfying feeling of satiation and well-being. The neurotic, on the other hand, not having found such satisfaction, may repeatedly seek it, yet find only frustration.

These cases are rare exceptions, however, and a spouse should be very cautious about drawing inferences of emotional disturbance from what may seem excessive demands. Most of these disputes can be reduced simply to a matter of one or both spouses refusing to love. And not just in sexual relations; their lack of loving is apparent in all areas of their marriage. For these couples, the solution should be obvious since it is also the essential foundation of the marriage—loving. Those couples, however, who cannot, even though motivated by love, seem to achieve a mutually satisfactory adjustment in their love-making should not hesitate to seek professional counseling to aid them in overcoming what can become a corrosive area of disagreement.

FRIGIDITY

Sexual frigidity is without doubt the greatest sexual problem threatening contemporary marriages. It is not an exaggeration to say that the majority of modern wives are, in some degree, frigid!

What this indicates in terms of unfulfilled marriages is appalling. And its frequency, if we are to judge by what we see happening to men and women, will probably increase. At a diagnostic staff meeting recently, a female patient, married and the mother of three, was interviewed by the staff psychiatrists and psychologists. During the discussion which followed, mention was made of the patient's symptoms of frigidity. A senior staff member shook his head and shrugged. "We probably can quit noting that as a symptom and just assume that these women are frigid, since most of them are!"

If the majority of wives are frigid, most of them are also unaware of their frigidity. They may feel that their marriage falls somehow short of the ideal union, but they haven't recognized either their frigidity or the attitudes which cause it.

Frigidity is defined as the inability to attain complete sexual fulfillment. This is not, however, the popular definition. Most couples we have talked with believe a frigid woman is totally lacking in sexual responsiveness, that she feels "nothing," or that she experiences pain and/or revulsion during intercourse. Defined this way, most wives are able to reject any suggestion of frigidity. But viewed correctly, frigidity is on a continuum which ranges from the extreme just described (usually termed "sexual anesthesia"), to a sexual responsiveness in which the wife is almost always able to reach orgasm during sexual relations. This is, admittedly, using a broader concept of frigidity than many writers employ, and it is for this reason that the incidence of frigidity among married women has been estimated by some to be as low as 10 per cent.

By our definition, a wife may achieve orgasm each time she has intercourse and yet still be frigid, since it isn't just the orgasm *per se* but the *kind* of orgasm which is important. A woman might, for example, reach a climax through masturbation and yet derive no satisfaction from intercourse. In such case, we would say she is frigid.

Earlier, we distinguished between the so-called *vaginal* and *clitoral* orgasms. Frigidity is the inability to attain vaginal, or total, orgasm. It is almost always psychological in origin; physical causes of the problem are so rare as to be nearly nonexistent. Contrary to popular belief, frigidity is seldom, if ever, caused by inept sexual technique, nor can it be cured by employing new skills or variations. The old canard "there are no frigid women, only inadequate husbands" is patently false. There *are* frigid women, many of them, and the most skilled lovers would be powerless to "cure" them.

A problem as complex as frigidity can't be given anything approaching proper treatment in a chapter. We can do no more than touch on the genesis of the problem: resentment toward men, negative maternal influence, antisexualism, and all the learned attitudes and responses which make it difficult if not impossible to make a total commitment. If the wife recognizes this, however, she has taken the first step toward eliminating it. She must keep in mind two very important points: first, her problem began long before she married, and only if she works to change her attitudes will the problem be relieved; and second, frigidity is far more than a *sexual* problem.

Some women may find help in reading *The Power of*

Sexual Surrender by Marie N. Robinson, M.D. (Doubleday & Company, Inc., 1959). Dr. Robinson gives an insightful picture of the problem of frigidity, its causes, and cure, and in a highly readable style. Even if a wife is convinced that this is not her problem, we recommend the book as "must" reading. The author gives a detailed description of the ideal woman which every wife, seeking to achieve happiness in her marriage, would do well to keep before her.

We have done no more than briefly describe the most frequently encountered sexual problems. In some cases, patience, understanding, and above all, love will enable a couple to work through the difficulty. If the problem persists, however, they should seek help. In any case, the obligation to strive for growth in their marriage makes it imperative that they not permit the condition to go unheeded. Listening to the advice of friends and relatives, however, will seldom help, and it may make things worse. Only a competent psychiatrist or clinical psychologist is qualified to counsel a couple with such problems.

CHAPTER XIII

Toward Growth in Sexual Love

WE CAN'T BUILD a good marriage without a good model to follow. But since most marriages we see fall far short of the Christian ideal, we may make a serious mistake if we choose someone else's marriage as our model.

Most husbands and wives employ their parents' marriages as their model. Since it is usually the only marriage they have observed at close range, they take it as the prototype of all marriage. As a result, they build a marriage which may be no worse than their parents', but is certainly no better. If we are looking toward a successful marriage, not one in which the spouses merely tolerate each other and somehow manage to co-exist, we would do well to critically evaluate—and probably reject—these models and their influence. We should ask ourselves, and each other, if these marriages represent what we hope our marriage will become.

We should turn the same critical eye on the marriages of our friends. If we don't, we may incorporate these models as criteria of a good marriage, and we may also expose ourselves to the corrosive environment of cynicism and bitterness. Morning coffee klatches, cocktail parties, and even meetings of parish organizations are often settings in which nothing other than marital failure is witnessed. Unless this is recognized, and guarded against, a couple may, without awareness, settle for the same "second best."

When we married, we had no clear notion of what marriage could, or should, be, only some idea of what we did not want our marriage to become. Over the years, we have learned much. We have found that truly beautiful Christian marriages do exist, albeit they are too few. We have learned that a mysterious and transcending "oneness" can develop.

Perhaps most important, we discovered that the model to be followed must be constructed by husband and wife: it must be their ideal of perfection.

This is our description of a *good* marriage:

1   *The marriage is built on a firm set of values and convictions which are shared by husband and wife. These convictions give meaning and purpose to their life. They know what they believe in and they are in complete accord in the principles which they follow. Their marriage is directed toward God and centered in Christ.*

2   *They are fully cognizant of their respective sexual roles and identities. He has a mature understanding of what it means to be a husband and father; she knows what she is to become as a wife. Both of them find deep satisfaction in their roles.*

3   *Communication is excellent. Not just good, but excellent. And they each continually work to improve it.*

4   *Both can say with honesty that each year of their marriage has been better than the year before, that it has become more romantic, more exciting, and more meaningful.*

5   *They are not attempting to mold or change each other. He finds many things in himself which he strives to change; she is aware of undesirable and unloving habits*

in herself which she works to eliminate; but they don't fall into the fatal error of making their love conditional upon change in the one to whom they are wed. Thus, they avoid that dangerous IF which makes love provisional: "If only he (or she) would change . . ."

6 *At no time have either of them had any regrets. While they may recognize that not all are called to the vocation of marriage, the joy they have found together makes them feel somewhat sorry for their single friends.*

7 *They at all times witness their marriage. Those who know them find it difficult to think of them individually; to think of one, is to think of both. The fulfillment they have found compels them to talk of their marriage, to virtually shout the good news from the rooftops. In doing so, they very effectively "show forth Christ."*

This is not a description of the ideal, although many disillusioned and cynical couples will view our description as idealistic. Why? Because it seems so far removed from *their* reality? We have repeated this description many times to groups as well as couples we have counseled. And most often it elicits skepticism. We have repeatedly been asked to estimate the number of couples who can claim to have experienced what we describe as a good marriage. Our answer: perhaps one in a hundred. Or maybe even this is an optimistic guess. But this hardly seems to be the more important question. The issue is whether or not such a marriage is possible of attainment by most. Our answer can only be an unequivocal YES. Since God called us to this vocation, to suggest that only a "chosen few" can find fulfillment in it is to infer that God is unjust. Christ himself spoke of it as a union in which two become one. He promises the grace necessary to reach this goal. We flatly reject the implication that He would deny this to all but a few.

Furthermore, we know such a marriage is possible. How? First of all, we have found it in our own marriage. Every year it has seemed that God has revealed more of the mysterious beauty of this sacrament to us. Every day He has shown us ever more of the continual honeymoon that the life to which He has called us can become. And how do we account for this? Did we each have ideal backgrounds? Or exceptional training and instruction in marriage? Or compatibility of interests? Hardly. We too were subjected to the pervasive cynicism of society. We heard all the dire predictions about the honeymoon coming to an end, about marriage being a fifty-fifty proposition, about it having its ups and downs, about it being no "bed of roses." We had seen no ideal marriage, nor even any which we could say fit our description of a *good* marriage. Marriage was presented as a relationship perpetuated by a never-ending series of compromises, a sort of "getting along together" and "sticking it out" through a tedious "thick and thin." We had no answer for the cynics then. We could only cling to a vague dream and meet their predictions of doom with silence. "Just wait until you've been married five years (or seven, or ten, or some other magical number)," they said. "Wait until you have four or five children." "Wait until you have bills you can't meet." Well, we waited. We didn't believe them then, but we had no answer to meet the weight of their unhappy experience. Now we do. Now you might say we have outlasted and outnumbered the criteria of their predictions. They have our sympathy and our prayers, but not our concordance. Now we can raise our voices. We can and do say to those entering this vocation: "Don't settle for less. Don't listen to the cynics. Cling to your ideal. Pray together. You can have a marriage beyond the beauty of your dreams."

And to you who have lost the dream, you husbands and

wives who have become disillusioned and cynical: this has not been our experience alone. We have seen marriages just like yours begin to grow; we have seen them rise like a Phoenix from the ashes and reach the transcendent heights of a fulfilling Christian marriage. These are couples who have made the choice of loving in all that it encompasses. Such a marriage is yours for the loving.

We have spoken of love as a "giving of self," but this definition is inadequate just as all definitions of love must be inadequate. Love is a mystery. It is not analyzable. Nor can it be conditional or judgmental. To ask why we love another is meaningless. If it is love, we do not love another *because* of their attributes nor *despite* their failings; we love the *person*. To desire change in them or to accept them only partially is to fail in loving.

We said our description was not the ideal. It can't be, since such a *good* marriage is attainable and the ideal of perfection can never be attained. But in continually striving for perfection in our marriage we will find such a *good* marriage.

We have discovered a very good test of a good marriage. Ask a couple: "Who gives the most in your marriage?" In a *good* marriage, the answer is always the same from both. They are each firmly convinced that the one to whom they are married is giving more than they are.

You may have noticed, we didn't mention sexual compatibility in our description. Having read this far, the reasons are probably apparent. Barring certain physical problems, if a couple can describe their marriage in the words of our outline, you can be sure their sexual relations will be not merely good but wonderful. We flatly deny that any couple can have a satisfactory sexual relationship, one that is everything it should be, unless the whole marriage is good.

Throughout these chapters, we have emphasized the

need for communication. Now we would like to expand what we have said. Lack of communication is by far the most common complaint of couples, much more prevalent than sexual problems. They complain of unwillingness to converse, incompatibility of interests, and repeated misunderstandings. But what do they mean when they talk of "communication"?

In order to love, we must have a knowledge of the loved one; we must know, on far more than a superficial level, the feelings, needs, and desires of the one to whom we are joined. This should be what is meant by communication. But more often than not, the spouse who complains of a lack of communication is speaking only of a frustrated desire for conversation—or the inability to "make a point."

Good communication is a high goal, and one not easily reached. To tell a couple they should strive to communicate is seldom of much help. Communication is a skill and, like all skills, must be learned. But this won't happen overnight; nor will it be learned effortlessly or painlessly. Nevertheless, it is a skill which can be acquired—and must, if the marriage is to mature. It implements all which we described as a good marriage.

So many factors may act to hinder communication that it becomes a matter of wonder that humans can communicate as well as they do, which isn't really well at all. Take, for example, our use of language. Words simply do not convey the same meaning to all, and hence don't elicit the same reactions from all. The problem isn't one of inadequate vocabulary or imprecise word usage, but differences in the associations we learn to various words. The word "love" is a good example. To most people, the words "I love you" express positive feelings of warmth, and affection. We enjoy being told, "I love you" by the one to whom we are closest. And yet experiences may result in a far different reaction. Let us suppose that during childhood the individual heard these words many times from a tyrannical father or a rejecting mother. We might then expect a far different reaction, one of mistrust and cynicism: "I don't believe you really love me, so don't say it."

We each carry into marriage countless associations to various words, associations which may vary greatly from those of our spouses. But this alone would not necessarily create a problem were it not that these differences in meaning and association are so seldom clarified. Instead, couples tend to make a mistake which is fatal to communication. They assume that they each have the same associations. That is, they each immediately conclude that they *know* what the other one is attempting to say. And, without any further clarification, they respond, each within his or her own frame of reference and each assuming the other has the same frame of reference.

As a result, even a compliment may be interpreted as an insult. A couple we spoke with recently told us of an argument they had which proved a classic example of this. She was wearing a new dress when her husband arrived home from work. He stepped back, and looked at her admiringly, "I like it. It's a good color on you and the stripes add to it." That did it! His wife turned on her heel and stalked from the room, and for the remainder of the evening she refused to speak. Her reaction might appear totally irrational and without provocation, but let's look at it. For several months, she had been gaining weight, not a great deal, nor even enough to be noticeable to her husband. But she was painfully aware of it. To her, the addition of a few pounds meant the loss of her youthful figure. To her chagrin, she found her wardrobe no longer fit, and it was this discovery which prompted her purchase of the dress. She selected vertical stripes because she felt they would have a slimming effect. This was her association to the stripes. Hence, when her husband commented on the attractiveness of the stripes, she interpreted it as a "dig" at her for being overweight. She was so painfully aware of her weight problem that she projected her feelings to her husband and interpreted them as his reaction. She was convinced that this was what he meant by the compliment.

Couples fall into this error time and time again. If only we would learn to clarify what we say to each other and to pause long enough to make certain we understand fully what the other one means, many misunderstandings might be avoided. In this instance, the wife had mentally added several additional remarks to her husband's compliment so that what she "heard" was something such as, "I'm glad you selected a striped dress; it doesn't make you appear quite as fat as you are," a thought which had never entered his mind.

Breakdown in communication also results from the all too common practice of interpreting facial expressions and voice inflections. It is a mistake made by nearly all of us. We explain our reactions by saying, "It isn't so much what he said, but the tone in his voice when he said it," or, "I could tell how she felt from the look on her face." The fact is, facial expression and voice inflection are very poor means of communication, very poor indeed. We are seldom able to accurately and consistently interpret either. This is just as true of husbands and wives, even though we may think otherwise. How many times have we experienced something like this: The husband arrives home from work. His wife has had a particularly exhausting day, and her face reflects her tiredness. He interprets her expression, however, as one of annoyance or rejection, and he reacts to it: "What's wrong?" "Nothing," she answers. "Yes, there is. I can see it in your face. Now tell me what's wrong."

Her answer is the same. Usually the same question and answer are repeated several times, to the increasing annoyance of both. In these cases, both are to blame; the husband, for leaping to an interpretation of her facial expression, and the wife, for not telling him of her fatigue.

We don't deny communication can take many forms other than words; facial expression, bodily movement, and voice inflection may, of course, communicate feelings, but, as we pointed out in Chapter VIII, words are still best —*provided we strive to clarify the meaning of the words we employ.*

With many couples, communication has been virtually extinguished. They claim they can find nothing to discuss. With one couple this had become such a problem that they asked for a list of suggested topics to help them get started conversing—after eleven years of marriage! This is the pet peeve of countless wives; their husbands just simply don't talk to them. The time they spend together is filled with silence, interrupted only rarely by the most superficial observations on children, family finances, and the trivia which fill their day-by-day existence. In most cases, the situation worsens over time; each year they communicate less. They'll admit they had no difficulty conversing during their courtship. Why then do they find it increasingly difficult the longer they live together and the more they know of each other?

It is specifically that they *have* learned so much of each other. It gives rise to the element of *threat*. As they learn more about each other, they become increasingly threatened, and they increasingly do and say things which threaten the other one. They learn the Achilles heel of their spouse, the areas of greatest vulnerability. Even though this may be unintended, in time, every conversation becomes potentially threatening, even the most innocuous. If then one or both are insecure—and made to feel even more insecure—the added fear may bring on this defensive withdrawal into a shell of silence.

Biblical writers used the word "knowing" in reference to sexual relations; they spoke of "knowing" man, or "knowing" woman, and a very fitting description it is. We reveal ourselves in our sexual union, and if we are to love each other fully, we must know each other fully; we must be able to communicate our sexual needs and feelings. But if communication generally is difficult for a couple, discussion of sexuality may be nearly impossible. It goes right to the core of what we are as men and women; nothing could be more revealing—or frightening if we are insecure. This is so not only of discussion of sexuality in the narrow sense, the marital union, but also of sexuality in the broadest meaning of the word: our sexual roles and identity.

On the whole, men are more threatened than their wives by discussion of their sexual relationship. In fact, many husbands are reluctant to engage in serious conversation with their wives if it touches on anything "personal."

Not that men alone are capable of being threatened. But because of the masculine role of leadership, they are more often, and more easily, threatened sexually. Women are more often threatened in other areas, but no less so. When we speak of threat, we are talking about something, a stimulus, that is, which is capable of arousing fear, and which causes us to defend ourselves. But it is usually more complex than simply a conditioned association of stimulus-response à la Pavlov's conditioning the salivary response in dogs. In a social interaction, there is an intervening variable between the stimulus and the response of fear. We call it *verbal mediation*.

Verbal mediation is itself a response to the stimulus. It then, in turn, acts as a stimulus to elicit an emotional response (e.g., fear). It is what the individual tells himself about a given situation (the stimulus). For example, one young man in his twenties suffered such severe anxiety when faced with new social situations that he avoided nearly all opportunities to join with others. He had never gone out on a date, had never accepted an invitation to a party, and had been unable, because of his fear, to walk in and apply for a job. It was not other persons, per se, however, which raised this anxiety, but his feelings of inadequacy, and the "instructions" he repeatedly gave himself. ("If I say or do something out of place, they will ridicule me and think I am a fool, and this will be a terrible, irreparable calamity; I'll be emotionally *destroyed!*")

In the area of sexuality, most anxiety involves such verbal mediation. Unless husband and wife are on guard, almost any sexual words or actions by the other one may set off a verbally mediated chain reaction resulting in anxiety. And anxiety crushes effective communication. Therefore, in order for communication between spouses to develop, especially if they are to understand their sexuality and grow in sexual love, they must realize that expression by the other one of sexual feelings and desires—or even lack of them—is seldom either an attack or a challenge. Unless they do, they will repeatedly feel threatened; every word they exchange will carry surplus meanings which can only serve to pull them further apart, meanings which they each supply through verbal mediation.

So many of our reactions are egocentric. We are so very afraid of being rejected, of being thought stupid, or immature, or bad, or in some way inadequate. We build walls about ourselves which keep us from being touched by others. And which keep us from touching others. Ultimately, these walls emotionally smother us. They become part of an illness which pervades our society. Men and women complain of loneliness and of being unloved, but *isolation* is a better word for it than loneliness. The fear, almost terror, of being hurt prevents them from ever getting close to another human being, one probably as afraid as themselves.

The first move in breaking down these walls is a critical analysis of our thinking. In this self-appraisal, the questions should center on "What am I telling myself about this situation, or about what he or she said, or about what they will be thinking of me?" And then the next question: "Does what I am telling myself, and the conclusions I am drawing, make sense; is there any sound reason for feeling this threatened?"

The questions may be specific to what we find threatening. "If my wife tells me she didn't reach an orgasm, does it make any sense for me to feel that I am a failure as a man?" "If he failed to respond amorously even though I wore my filmiest negligee, did it really prove he doesn't love me?" "When she asked me to empty the trash, was she really treating me as a child and playing the role of my mother, or was it my own feeling of immaturity?" Developing the habit of asking such questions and striving to answer them on the basis of what we *know* to be so, rather than on quickly drawn inferences, may do much to dissolve the blocks which impede communication.

Most important we must have the desire to communicate, the desire to know and understand this person. In other words, the desire to love. With this as their motive, husband and wife will be willing to undergo what may be a painful and perhaps frightening period during which they struggle to find a freedom of communication. For a time, this may mean forcing themselves to talk, even when it is very uncomfortable. And it will mean permitting the other one to freely express feelings and thoughts which may be threatening, and resisting the temptation to counterattack.

This self-analysis of our verbal mediations should be

part of an overall attempt to know ourselves and understand who and what we are. This is a tedious process, one which demands that we each strip off the defenses behind which we hide. And make no mistake, we each have these protective layers. Only as we are able to peel them away, however, are we able to confront what we are and what we are to become. And only then are we able to relate fully to others, and to love them. The task is never finished. Each layer reveals the next layer and that one the next. But each time we learn more of ourselves, and discover more of loving.

Throughout this book we have used two words: *freedom* and *love*. Both words, we have found, are very disturbing to some, especially when they are employed in the context of morality in Christian marriage. They apparently think of morality as a restriction of freedom. In other words, they view sexual freedom as *license*.

But the freedom of which we are speaking, is the freedom which permits husband and wife to grow, together, in beauty and sanctity. It is a freedom from fear, from ignorance, from unwholesome attitudes, from scrupulosity, from bitterness and resentment. It is the freedom to *love*.

As this freedom grows, we discover more and more doors opening, an ever-increasing number of opportunities to love—more. Loving always has a way of bringing us to even greater depths of loving. The freedom is both the "freedom *to* sexually love" and the "freedom *of* sexual love." As we become free to love each other sexually, an entire horizon of marital love opens before us. It creates an atmosphere of love, an atmosphere of Christ.

Again we repeat, there are many failures along the way, both large and small. They seem almost daily. But, along with St. Paul, we can "glory in our infirmities" if we accept them as challenges to growth. For the final time: loving is not always easy—but it does become easier.

What seems like a long time ago, we found an examination of conscience, one particularly suited to marriage, one that can well be employed many times each day: "Have I loved? In what ways can I love more?"

Suggested Readings

ARNOLD, F. X. *Woman and Man*. New York: Herder and Herder, 1963.

BIRD, JOSEPH and LOIS. *Marriage Is for Grownups*. Garden City, N.Y.: Doubleday & Co., Inc., 1969.

FROMM, ERICH. *The Art of Loving*. New York: Harper & Row, 1956.

HÄRING, BERNARD. *Christian Marriage: A Way of Salvation*. Chicago: Christian Family Movement, 1963.

LEPP, IGNACE. *The Psychology of Loving*. Baltimore: Helicon Press, 1963.

LUNDBERG, FERDINAND and FARNHAM, MARYNIA F. *Modern Woman: The Lost Sex*. New York: Harper & Bros., 1947.

ROBINSON, MARIE N. *The Power of Sexual Surrender*. Garden City, N.Y.: Doubleday & Co., Inc., 1959.